T0345198

APPLIED SOCIOLOGY OF HEALTH AND ILLNESS

This popular and accessible text continues to cover the basic principles of the sociology of health and illness in an eminently readable way. This fully revised second edition has been inspired, informed, and reviewed by medical students. By creatively employing a problem-based learning approach, the book examines commonly covered topics integrating underlying principles and research findings through real-life stories. The book investigates the relevance of sociology and considers a new direction – one that places sociology in the context of healthcare settings, making the topic more realistic, useful, and memorable.

The book will be an invaluable companion for medical students throughout undergraduate studies and is also a useful reference for students in nursing, social work, psychology, and sociology, as well as qualified doctors and healthcare practitioners.

Applied Sociology of Health and Illness

A Problem-Based Learning Approach

Second Edition

Costas S. Constantinou
Professor of Medical Sociology
University of Nicosia Medical School
Nicosia, Cyprus

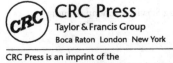

CRC Press
Taylor & Francis Group
Boca Raton London New York

CRC Press is an imprint of the
Taylor & Francis Group, an **informa** business

Second edition published 2023
by CRC Press
6000 Broken Sound Parkway NW, Suite 300, Boca Raton, FL 33487-2742

and by CRC Press
4 Park Square, Milton Park, Abingdon, Oxon, OX14 4RN

CRC Press is an imprint of Taylor & Francis Group, LLC

© 2023 Costas S. Constantinou

First edition published by CRC Press 2014

This book contains information obtained from authentic and highly regarded sources. While all reasonable efforts have been made to publish reliable data and information, neither the author[s] nor the publisher can accept any legal responsibility or liability for any errors or omissions that may be made. The publishers wish to make clear that any views or opinions expressed in this book by individual editors, authors or contributors are personal to them and do not necessarily reflect the views/opinions of the publishers. The information or guidance contained in this book is intended for use by medical, scientific or health-care professionals and is provided strictly as a supplement to the medical or other professional's own judgement, their knowledge of the patient's medical history, relevant manufacturer's instructions and the appropriate best practice guidelines. Because of the rapid advances in medical science, any information or advice on dosages, procedures or diagnoses should be independently verified. The reader is strongly urged to consult the relevant national drug formulary and the drug companies' and device or material manufacturers' printed instructions, and their websites, before administering or utilizing any of the drugs, devices or materials mentioned in this book. This book does not indicate whether a particular treatment is appropriate or suitable for a particular individual. Ultimately it is the sole responsibility of the medical professional to make his or her own professional judgements, so as to advise and treat patients appropriately. The authors and publishers have also attempted to trace the copyright holders of all material reproduced in this publication and apologize to copyright holders if permission to publish in this form has not been obtained. If any copyright material has not been acknowledged please write and let us know so we may rectify in any future reprint.

ISBN: 9781032188669 (hbk)
ISBN: 9781032188652 (pbk)
ISBN: 9781003256687 (ebk)

DOI: 10.1201/9781003256687

Typeset in Sabon
by Deanta Global Publishing Services, Chennai, India

To my family

Contents

Foreword to the first edition

WHY MEDICAL SOCIOLOGY IS IMPORTANT
FOR A MODERN MEDICAL EDUCATION

It was September 2006 when I first started teaching sociology, or better, medical sociology, to medical students at the then newly established Norwich Medical School at the University of East Anglia. I had taken up this important role before doing research on women's experience of severe chronic illness and on patients' understanding of informed consent in experiential medical trials. I remember being very excited at finally having been given the chance to contribute to the education of a new generation of doctors who surely would all be very fascinated in what I had to tell them about the social aspects of medicine and the importance of taking patients' life stories and their often-complex backgrounds into account. Surely everybody would agree with me, so I thought, that medicine was not just about the body, but also about the person, their ideas, their experiences, and their view on being a patient. Surely, I thought, everybody would also agree with me that modern medicine also needed to take into account that for medical treatment to be successful, the doctors would have to be very much aware of their own social background as well as that of the patient. So, I set out to design the curriculum. To my astonishment, not only was there hardly anything published on how to teach medical sociology to medical students, but it was also the case that the lecturers who taught medical sociology before I did – all medical professionals – thought it was all just common-sense understanding. The first year of integrating medical sociology into a modern medical education I was torn, on the one hand, between medical professionals who thought that anybody with a little bit of interest in 'the social' could do my job, and on the other hand students, who feared that they would never be able to satisfy my theoretical interest. I thus asked myself: is medical sociology all about an arcane theoretical knowledge that only a select few who had spent years studying it could understand? Or was it indeed all only 'common-sense knowledge' and I had grossly overrated all the theoretical ideas that underpinned a theoretical model of how societies organise curing, healing, and caring? In supervising students, who were worried that they might not satisfy my theoretical demands, I often found myself saying that an explanation of the social facts would suffice and that I would not expect them to know the difference between Karl Marx and Anthony Giddens. In order not to make my classes seem too complicated and difficult for students of medicine, who after all were not social scientists, I cut out most of the theoretical background. Even though my task was to rewrite the curriculum, I had to stick to lecture titles that had already been designed by my predecessor who had left the post two years before my arrival because the timetables had already been written for the commencing academic year. I had read the feedback that students gave about the lectures in sociology before my arrival, and they had even said that they felt sociology was, after all, just 'common sense'. I was thus torn between wanting to demonstrate that sociology is not as 'esoteric' as some students feared, nor that it was just common sense. There was certainly a need for further literature research on how sociology should be taught in medical education.

THE MEDICAL CURRICULUM

The other challenge I encountered was that there was not yet a template curriculum for teaching sociology in a medical school. Three years after I started my lectureship, the UK's General Medical Council (GMC) published *Tomorrow's Doctors* (2009), which discusses in general what a newly qualified medical professional should know and gives the social sciences equal weighting with the natural sciences, yet there were still no guidelines for social science teaching in medicine. Most textbooks of medical sociology, with a few exceptions (e.g., Iphofen and Poland, 1998), were written for sociology departments that teach medical sociology within the context of a sociology department. I also felt that because of the way the sociology lectures were integrated into the overall curriculum, there was a certain amount of deliberate simplification of highly complex sociological theories. Medical sociology was mostly seen as a handmaiden to medicine, as an explanation for human behaviour in health and illness and giving guidelines on how to improve adherence to the medical paradigm. Medicine starts out with a 'medical problem' and then seeks a social explanation for it (see Browner, 1999). Medical sociology is thus conceptualised as commenting on established medical knowledge and human behaviour rather than as a critical comment on medicine as a social practice and a social construct per se. The second point of departure fundamentally challenges medical practice as it proposes that medicine, science, and technology are a social construct, contingent upon a specific culture and a specific society at any given time and place (Lock and Gordon, 1988). The challenge I faced was to design a curriculum that was at the same time founded in sociological theory and which conveyed the underlying axiom that medicine, disease concepts, illness behaviour, and curing were, after all, socially constructed. The presentation of this to the students should not come across as too radical but students should be made to reflect on their role as future doctors within this situation. It should also make sense to students who were not previously trained in sociology.

After systematically reviewing scholarly journals on medical education and sociology of medicine, it became clear that even though most medical schools in the UK now have full-time academically trained medical sociologists in their teams, there was little published research that scrutinised the impact on the discipline of sociology or medical education (Peters et al., 2006). Only one paper directly addressed the issue (Russell et al., 2004) and the findings were similar to my experience: the GMC places increasing importance on social science approaches to medical training, yet there was, and still is, no template curriculum. Most importantly, however, Russell et al. (2004) pointed out that social scientists had been marginalised in medical schools and most social scientists felt that their role within a medical school did not allow them to exhibit and explore their most treasured professional identity: their theoretical prowess. As the authors put it, there is a

> recognized tension between what academic social and behavioural scientists might regard as core content – fundamental topics that it would be essential to cover in any introductory course – within their own disciplines, and what they would identify as core topics and approaches needed to train the kind(s) of doctor ideally required in the UK today.
>
> *(Russell et al., 2004, p. 412)*

I thus faced the challenge of designing a curriculum without a template and without being able to draw on debates within the discipline of medical sociology. Research in the journal *Social Science & Medicine,* the flagship journal of medical sociology, argued that medical sociology seems not to have taken on the challenge of engaging outside its own ivory tower. Clair et al. (2007) show that most publications in journals such as *Social Science & Medicine* and the *Journal of Health and Social Behaviour* shy away from engaging with public policy and giving recommendations on how to improve healthcare. There is a dearth of applied recommendations, as the authors put it. I suggest there is a similar tendency when it comes to discussing applied sociology teaching in medical schools.

It is with this background in mind that I am so grateful to Costas Constantinou for having finally filled the gap between these two positions and for presenting us with a blueprint on how to teach medical sociology within modern, problem-based learning (PBL) medical education. Medical teaching delivered through PBL, i.e., a system in which weekly scenarios with specific themes requires students to research the topics and teach themselves, is a challenge in itself because it seems to bridge another gap: that of the 'two cultures', i.e., the humanities and the natural sciences. The discipline of medicine in itself is always considered as bridging this gap. As C.P. Snow (1959) famously argued in his elaborations on our modern academic structure, our way of understanding the world is divided into 'two cultures': the humanities and the basic sciences. Snow's distinction had described the status quo, yet at the same time created a situation in which the humanities and social sciences were defined as contesting the reality we live in as a construct, whereas the basic sciences work on the principle that good science discovers this reality. According to Snow, medicine is part of the category of scientists who believe in the progress of society through science, technology, and industry, whereas the second, to which sociology belongs, is a culture of 'literary intellectuals' who believe in the 'social construction of reality' and who are 'natural Luddites', critical in their assessment of advanced industrialised societies. The history of the two disciplines also reflects this distinction: even though European medicine has its origin as one of the 'artes liberales', modern medicine is very much based on the pillars of scientific reasoning (Good, 1994). Western medicine distinguishes itself from other medical systems by being built on the heritage of dissection. The cutting open of the dead body brought knowledge into what was previously purely based on belief and assumption. However, this heritage created the paradigm of 'seeing is believing', of disorder and distress rooted in anatomy, an imbalance in bodily chemistry and, finally, genetic determinism.

Contrary to medicine, sociology, especially medical sociology, is a relatively new discipline. Annandale and Field (2001) describe how medical sociology in Britain was consolidated, after some struggles in the late 1960s and early 1970s, with the foundation of the journal *Sociology of Health and Illness*, which is now recognised as a major international journal in the field. They point out that by the end of the 1990s, there were 47 full-time professors of medical sociology in UK Higher Education departments, as opposed to 10 at the end of the 1980s. Annandale and Field describe British medical sociology as constituted by a core concern with the experience of health and illness, an interest in health inequalities which are a product of social class, gender, ethnicity, and age, and the provision of healthcare (2001, p. 249). Anthony Giddens, for example, defines a sociologist as a professional who is able to 'break free from the immediacy of personal circumstances and put things into a wider context' (1991, p. 4). He refers to the American sociologist C. Wright Mills, who coined the term 'the sociological imagination', by which he meant the ability to 'think ourselves away' from the familiar routines of our daily lives in order to look at them anew (ibid.). This micro-perspective, however, allows us to see many events that seem to concern the individual alone as being part of a bigger picture. Giddens cites the example of someone who decides to go and drink a cup of coffee: a sociologist could observe the ritual of drinking coffee, the communication it engenders in the office environment, the idea of having spare time (individual and group behaviour), and the idea of coffee production and commerce (globalisation) and how this then influences someone's decision to choose 'normal' coffee or fairtrade coffee (consumption). Using this approach, a simple decision to go and consult a GP about a health concern could be analysed from the level of interaction, to self-help, to pharmaceutical power, and to institutionalisation of medical care.

In the GMC's guidelines to good medical education, *Tomorrow's Doctors*, the duties of a doctor registered with the GMC are outlined. They point out that in order to have a good relationship with patients, the content of what future doctors need to know is different to what they had to know in the past. Future doctors not only need to know and understand the rights of patients, but also respect the diversity of patients (GMC, 2009, p. 15). This means that they should respect patients regardless of their lifestyle, culture, beliefs, race, colour, gender, sexuality, disability, age, or social or economic status.

However, this document also suggests that C.P. Snow's analysis of the two cultures is no longer applicable to the current relationship between social science (in our case sociology) and the natural sciences (in our case medicine). The GMC actively advocates the inclusion of the social science perspective in medical education. After all, in the ideal-type medicine and ideal-type sociology, both share a common interest: to understand and improve people's lives, their ailments and experiences (Bauman and Tester, 2001; Flyvbjerg, 2001). Costas Constantinou's book not only contributes to bridging the gap between theoretical sociology and medical education, it also contributes to the way we teach a new generation of students – how to understand patients in context, how to treat them with respect and, ultimately, how to be a better medical doctor.

Dr Andrea Stöckl
Lecturer, Sociology and Anthropology of Medicine
Team Leader, Sociology & Anthropology Module
University of East Anglia, Norwich

REFERENCES

Annandale E, Field D. Medical sociology in Great Britain. In: Cockerham WC, editor. *The Blackwell Companion to Medical Sociology*, pp. 246–262. Oxford: Blackwell Publishers; 2001.

Bauman Z, Tester K. *Conversations with Zygmunt Bauman*. Cambridge: Polity; 2001.

Browner C. On the medicalization of medical anthropology. *Med Anthropol Q.* 1999; 13(2): 135–40.

Clair JM, Cullen C, Hinote BP, Robinson CO, Wasserman JA. Developing, integrating, and perpetuating new ways of applying sociology to health, medicine, policy, and everyday life. *Soc Sci Med.* 2007; 64(1): 248–58.

Flyvbjerg B. *Making Social Science Matter: Why Social Inquiry Fails and How It Can Succeed Again*. Cambridge: Cambridge University Press; 2001.

Giddens A. *Modernity and Self-Identity. Self and Society in the Late Modern Age*. Stanford, CA: Stanford University Press; 1991.

General Medical Council. *Tomorrow's doctors*. London: GMC; 2009. Accessible online at www.gmc-uk.org/education/undergraduate/GMC_tomorrows _doctors.pdf.

Good B. *Medicine, Rationality and Experience*. Cambridge: Cambridge University Press; 1994.

Iphofen R, Poland F. *Sociology in Practice for Health Care Professionals*. Basingstoke: Macmillan; 1998.

Lock M, Gordon D. *Biomedicine Examined*. Dordrecht and London: Kluwer Academic Publishers; 1988.

Peters S, Livia A. Relevant behavioural and social science for medical undergraduates: A comparison of specialist and non-specialist educators. *Med Educ*. 2006; 40(10): 1020–6.

Russell A, van Teijlingen E, Lambert H, Stacy R. Social and behavioural science education in UK medical schools: Current practice and future directions. *Med Educ*. 2004; 38(4): 409–17.

Snow CP. *The Two Cultures*. Cambridge: Cambridge University Press; 1959.

Preface

In 1996, Steele and Marshall published an article in the journal *Teaching Sociology*, in which they described how sociology would evolve in terms of problem-solving in the decade that would follow. The authors highlighted that sociology already possessed the knowledge to understand and solve real social and individual problems and they thus anticipated a change. Similarly, certain scholars pointed out the benefits of experiential learning in sociology (DeMartini, 1983; Calderon and Farrell, 1996), while others wished to test the effectiveness of teaching sociology on the basis of problem-solving. For example, Lehman (1997, p. 72) wrote: 'I was struck by our [colleagues'] agreement that we wanted students to do sociology, to be able to use it, to employ a sociological perspective'. He continued, 'I was also struck by the confusion we shared about how to accomplish this'. Lehman (1997) subsequently employed problem-based learning (PBL) to help students learn more about gender stratification. He found that students learned better and developed a deeper understanding of the subject, remembered more, developed critical thinking, and learned how to research. In their attempt to prepare a course on the social history of American families, Ross and Hurlbert (2004) designed a PBL exercise in order to construct an environment for students to thoroughly discuss and critically approach the changing forms of the American family. About 70% of the students evaluated the exercise positively, 17% were uncertain, while 13% assessed the experience negatively. Some of those students who provided negative feedback indicated that they did not enjoy teamwork, while some others stated that the learning objectives were unclear. The authors considered, however, that given that 70% of students evaluated the PBL exercise positively, it could be considered as a successful approach. They concluded that PBL could be used to teach complex sociological issues.

More than ten years later, in their book, *Handbook of the Sociology of Medical Education*, Brosnan and Turner (2009) stressed that given the changes in types of diseases, morbidity, and healthcare, sociology could introduce new practical issues (e.g., disability, complementary, and alternative medicine, etc.) in medical education to inform medical curricula and medical practice. Interestingly in 2022, it seems that the gap between theoretical sociology and its use in applied medical settings remains, although the need for more applied sociology has been acknowledged and promoted in some relevant guidelines. For example, a report from the Behavioural & Social Sciences Teaching in Medicine (BeSST) Sociology Steering Committee included the core curriculum for sociology in the UK undergraduate medical education identified the importance of using clinical cases in order to clearly demonstrate the usefulness of sociology in understanding health and illness (Collett et al., 2016). In addition, Dikomitis et al. (2022) highlighted the importance of integrating sociology with medical education.

Having taught sociology and sociology of health and illness to medical, nursing, psychology, and social work students for almost 20 years, I was also faced with the difficulty of making sociology more practical and, thus, more useful to my students. I always included examples in my lectures, which helped students better understand the basic concepts. However, examples were mere snapshots and did not really account for the complexity of social reality. Thereafter, I looked for ways to make sociology more relevant to daily life, but it was not always clear how this could be achieved in a way that would be appealing to healthcare students.

Medical students at the University of Nicosia Medical School in Cyprus established the groundwork for achieving such a practical aspect of sociology, inspired the creation of both editions of this book, which relies on PBL, and informed refinement before publishing. The book applies the principles of PBL (Barrows, 1996) in the sense that all chapters start with a scenario and raise questions for students to discuss before they proceed. The scenario continues to unfold gradually, and sociological theories and principles are applied to explain the scenario that has been presented. As the scenario further unfolds, more issues are raised and additional sociological principles, theory, and research findings are used until the scenario comes to an end or the problem is solved.

How did students inspire and inform such an endeavour? It resulted from a combination of challenging the need for sociology, accidentally doing sociology, and reviewing an earlier version of the book. *First*, during one of the weekly review meetings, some students expressed concerns that it was difficult for them to understand why they had to have so many sessions in social sciences in order to become a doctor. They had a point. This is what triggered me to start thinking how to make sociology more usable. Students needed not just knowledge, but something more tangible to use in their practice. *Second*, it was during a period in 2012 when I was a PBL tutor for two modules in the first year of the medical programme and my students had initiated a discussion over a sociology learning objective that was not supposed to be covered in the PBL but had been covered during a lecture two days earlier. Students applied the main principles of the sociology of death to explain the case of a dying person and they shared the knowledge they acquired from the relevant lecture and discussed it thoroughly. They basically constructed a miniature sociology PBL session. I observed the session that the students constructed with great care and interest. It was then that I realised that there was a new direction in teaching sociology of health and illness to nurture and explore. The direction aimed at making sociology, as the cited scholars above had pointed out a few years ago, more practical, applicable, useful, and memorable. *Third*, when everything was put together and a draft prepared, students were invited to review the book. For the first edition published in 2014, fifteen students read parts of the book and provided feedback.

This second edition was also inspired by a medical student. Although I knew that the book had been used at some universities for teaching purposes, I was not sure how helpful it was for medical students until I received an email from a new medical student a couple of years ago. This new student wanted to thank me for having written such an appealing book for medical students. It was that email that enlightened me to initiate the process for preparing and publishing the second edition of this book. I followed the same procedure of drafting the book and collecting feedback from students. The second edition generated a lot more interest, resulting in 75 students reading one or more chapters and providing feedback by completing a questionnaire. On average, each chapter was reviewed by more than seven students. The questionnaire had eight closed questions to be rated on a scale from 1 (not at all) to 7 (a great deal) and two open questions for comments. The eighth question was about the overall grade and the scale was 1 (badly written) to 7 (excellent). The average scores on the closed questions showed that the chapters were scored similarly. The scores were: clarity of learning objectives (6.73), covering the learning objectives (6.66), comprehensible scenario (6.79), interesting scenario (6.43), clear sociological material (6.44), effective merging of the scenario with sociological material (6.55), usefulness for healthcare students and practitioners (6.55), and overall grade (6.44). Students were asked to make suggestions for improving the chapters; most of these suggestions were adopted. Also, students were asked to write a comment to promote the book, provided that their overall grade was higher than five. Students wrote very positive comments, some of which are found on the back cover of the book. To capture the essence of what I have just described in these last two paragraphs, this book has been inspired, informed, and reviewed by medical students. In other words, this book is a student-centred learning resource which has been developed by student feedback and it facilitates understanding by promoting engagement with the material (Constantinou, 2020).

In preparing the book, I had two important things in mind. *First*, I needed to cover the basic principles in the sociology of health and illness. *Second*, I had to write the scenarios or stories in such a way as to agree with the basic literature. The two (literature and scenarios) would need to merge together in a manner similar to the one experienced when watching a documentary that presented facts or observations supported by an explanatory commentary. To achieve this, I selected the most commonly covered topics in the sociology of health and illness, brought together the basic principles and research findings for each topic, and then wrote the stories in such a way as to fit the literature. I should say here that this was a demanding undertaking but a rewarding journey nonetheless as I had the opportunity to marry real-life stories with scientific knowledge.

Having clarified what the book is all about and how it was produced, I would now like to clarify what the book is not. *First*, the book is not a substitute for the existing textbooks in the sociology of health and illness. Instead, it offers a new way of applying and teaching the material; other textbooks could work as supplementary sources for further understanding the scenarios or cases that are presented in this book. By the same token, this book could work as a supplementary source for understanding the concepts and principles that are found in other textbooks. *Second*, the book is not about reducing sociology to individual cases, but the individual cases, which have been used to write the ten chapters of this book, work as examples of wider social trends in contemporary Western societies, and which I understand as plausible cases that health professionals could encounter in their daily practice.

The book's introduction presents Frank Bennet, a new medical student, who cannot understand why he has to attend so many sessions in sociology in order to become a doctor and, eventually, challenges the usefulness of sociology for medical practitioners. Frank engages in a long discussion with Dr Philip White, a teacher in his Sociology of Health and Illness class, in order to better understand the need for learning sociology. Motivated by Dr White, Frank then becomes immersed in the ten stories that this book presents and is expected to understand each one on the basis of sociological knowledge. He begins with Alem Parkins and her belief in the evil eye and ends with a patient, John Goodman, using digital health technology.

Costas S. Constantinou

REFERENCES

Barrows HS. Problem-based learning in medicine and beyond: A brief overview. In: Wilkerson L, Gijselaers WH, editors. *New Directions for Teaching and Learning*. San Francisco: Jossey-Bass Publishers; 1996, pp. 3–11.

Brosnan C, Turner BS. Introduction: The struggle over medical knowledge. In: Brosnan C, Turner BS, editors. *Handbook of the Sociology of Medical Education*. New York: Routledge; 2009, pp. 1–12.

Calderon J, Farrell B. Doing sociology: Connecting the classroom experience with a multiethnic school district. *Teach Sociol.* 1996; 24(1): 46–53.

Collett T, Brooks L, Forrest S, Harden J, Kelly M, Kendall K, MacBride-Stewart S, Sbaiti M, Stevenson F. A core curriculum for sociology in UK undergraduate medical education. *A Core Curriculum for Sociology in UK Undergraduate Medical Education*. 2016. Available at: https://www.besst.info/_files/ugd/3901ea_87ee230408434138b26135161bae60b9.pdf.

Constantinou CS. A reflexive GOAL framework for achieving student-centered learning in European higher education: From class learning to community engagement. *Societies* 2020; 10(4): 75.

DeMartini JR. Sociology, applied work, and experiential learning. *Teach Sociol.* 1983; 11(1): 17–31.

Dikomitis L, Wenning B, Ghobrial A, Adams KM. Embedding behavioural and social sciences across the medical curriculum: (Auto) ethnographic insights from medical schools in the United Kingdom. *Societies* 2022; 12: 101.

Lehman P. Group problem-solving approach to learning about gender stratification and research process in introductory sociology. *Teach Sociol.* 1997; 25: 72–77.

Ross S, Hurlbert JM. Problem-solving learning: An exercise on Vermont's legalization of civil unions. *Teach Sociol.* 2004; 32: 79–93.

Steele SF, Marshall S. On raising hopes of raising teaching: A glimpse of introduction to sociology in 2005. *Teach Sociol.* 1996; 24: 1–7.

Acknowledgements

Certainly, this book would not be a reality without the contribution of other people. I would therefore like to thank different people for different reasons. I would like to thank Professor Alexia Papageorgiou who encouraged me to turn a learning resource I had prepared for my PgCert into a book, Elisa Bosio for her patience to edit the language, Carrie Rodomar for her language editing and her useful comments and assistance with citations and referencing, Christina Loizou for her valuable expert feedback, Dimos Alekkou for his clinical psychology perspective, and Professor Peter McCrorie for his comments on the PBL style of the book. I would also like to thank Dr Andrea Stöckl, University of East Anglia, for her expert medical sociology feedback on a draft of the first edition of the book. An earlier version of the 2014 edition was reviewed by the following MBBS students at St George's, University of London (SGUL) Medical Programme delivered in Cyprus by the University of Nicosia Medical School: Melanie Dalton, Amy Lesner, Brian Richards, Sarah Anne Powell, Britain Baker, Christine Manuelian, Kevin Morrison, Jane Khalife, Yukari Blumenthal, Nisha Prasad, Samir Husainy, Georgios Kourounis, Patrick Tabet, Anna Lisa Gill, Christopher Veys.

An earlier version of the second edition of the book was reviewed and largely informed by feedback from 75 medical students registered in SGUL's MBBS programme, and the MD programme of the University of Nicosia Medical School, whom I thank greatly: Aasiya Syed, Aisha Yasmin Buba Bello, Ahmed Showry, Alex Ali Rezae, Aline Derlagen, Alma Sato, Anna Stark, Anthi Maria Lazaridi, Ao Shi, Arabella Maria

Constanza Borgstein, Basil Alawyia, Chani Rubinsohn, Christianna Balambanos, Christina Lee, Christine Bodine, Christopher William Raabe, Clemence Lagroy de Croutte, Deborah Temowo, Doaa Sallam, Emma Horiguchi, Emma Nordahl, Habib Mohamed, Hamreet Baidwan, Hosna Motamedian, Ioannis Apergis, Ioannis Karamatzanis, Julie Badawi-Najjar, Katerina Englezakis, Kaylee Briones, Khadijah Aliyu Aziz, Konstantina Damvakis, Konstantinos Kossenas, Kyle Alexander, Liranne Bitton, Lucinda Millsom, Maamoun Adra, Christina Fronista, Maria Issa, Maria Witkowiak, Mariam Hamam, Marianne Atieh, Marie Michele Macaron, May Yousef Hasan Hajeir, Mikhail Petritsym, Mira Azar, Nada Elbastawisi, Natalia Kritikou, Neha Najeeb, Olesia Verstiuk, Ornella Nohra, Ovidia Stray-Pedersen, Prakriti Sachdev, Petronella Johanna Van Heerden, Nicole Kolydas, Ramy Samia, Reem Fakak, Reem Matar, Roulla Panteli, Safa'a Khorshed Mohammed, Sara Al Zoubi, Shirin Akil, Sobhan Motamedian, Sotirios Gklegles, Stephania Christodoulou, Stephanie Kahura, Stylianos Rallidis, Stephen Matthew Ying-Fung Chui, Teranne Morrison, Toby Newton, Thomas Tavos, Vanessa Chow, Umamenan Kannathasan, Valeria Antoniou, Yael Cohen, Zoi Savva.

About the author

Costas S. Constantinou is Professor of Medical Sociology at the University of Nicosia Medical School, Cyprus. He holds a BA in psychology and sociology from Simon Fraser University in Canada, a MA in sociology from the University of Nicosia in Cyprus, and a PhD in social anthropology from the University of Bristol in the UK. He also holds a PgCert in Healthcare and Biomedical Education from St George's, University of London, UK. His research interests are illness experience, cultural competence, student-centred learning, teaching medical sociology, ageing, and qualitative research methodology.

Note about language

All names used in the chapter scenarios of this book are pseudonyms, and the scenarios are the result of the author's imagination. Any similarities between the scenarios and real-life stories are coincidental.

Introduction

....

WHY SOCIOLOGY OF HEALTH AND ILLNESS?

It is the beginning of a new academic year, and the first-year medical students visit the university for the induction week. All of the students appear to be excited and proud to have been accepted at the medical school in order to pursue their studies, and later a career, in medicine. They chat among themselves, meet faculty members, and review the curriculum once more so that everything is clear to them before they start their classes. In a related session, the course director, Professor Carol Simpson, presents the curriculum in detail; she reviews the basic and clinical sciences components first and then carries on presenting the social sciences. The social sciences are represented by psychology, epidemiology, sociology, research methods, communication skills, and ethics. One student, Frank Bennet, raises his hand in order to make a comment and Professor Carol nods at him:

Professor Carol: Yes, please.
Frank: I don't understand why we have so many sessions in social sciences subjects. We are here to learn how to become doctors, not social analysts!
Professor Carol: You are right. In the future you will be practising doctors and that is why you need to know about the social aspects of health.
Frank: I understand that epidemiological knowledge, statistics, medical ethics, communication with patients, and so on, are indeed helpful.

DOI: 10.1201/9781003256687-1

However, it is not clear to me why I should know about sociology, which is a largely theoretical discipline.

Professor Carol: I think that this is a good opportunity for our sociologist, Dr Philip White, to explain the importance of studying sociology within the medical programme.

Dr Philip: Good morning. Sociology is considered a requirement by many national medical councils around the world. However, we don't teach it simply because it is a requirement; rather, we teach sociology because it is very useful to medical practitioners.

Frank: I don't understand how this can be the case.

Dr Philip: We don't merely teach the general principles of sociology. Rather, we apply these general principles to health and illness. Sociology is the study of social relations, social groups, the structure of society, and the relationship between all of these. So, we basically try to examine the social aspects of health and illness, which means, for example, the social relations experienced within a health setting, the changes in people's social life due to a chronic condition, the influence of societies on people's way of understanding health and illness, and so forth.

Frank: Could you please be more specific? Perhaps you could provide an example of how sociology can be applied to health and illness?

Dr Philip: There are many areas in the sociology of health and illness but let me focus on a few important ones. These are: lay health beliefs, the body as a social construction, how people experience chronic diseases, labelling and stigma, social aspects of mental illness, social inequalities in health, gender and health, ethnic background and health, health and ageing, and digital health.

Frank: These are general areas. How can they be of use to medical students or doctors?

> *At this point, Dr Philip is slightly concerned that it might take a significant amount of time to explain how sociology can assist medical students and doctors; however, he decides to grasp the opportunity to elaborate on the matter as other students may have similar queries.*

Dr Philip: Doctors treat patients, correct? Patients are not dolls or objects, though; they are human beings who carry within them the values of the society they grew up in. This means that their thoughts and behaviours have been influenced by the social values they have been socialised with. If you, as doctors, know more about the social values that have influenced your patients, you could certainly understand more about their attitudes towards health, their health behaviour, and adherence to medication and treatment.

Frank: Surely, all patients wish to be well and will follow the medical treatment prescribed to them! I don't need to understand their processes of thought in order to perform my job.

Dr Philip: One would think so; however, in actuality, this is not always the case! Patients develop their own theories and understanding of health and do not always agree with their doctors. What would you do, for example, if you had a patient who had a stroke but did not accept your diagnosis? What would you do if the patient thought that it was the evil eye that had caused the problem, a belief the patient might carry from their home country?

Frank: I don't think that I would spend much time dealing with such issues. If the patient does not accept my medical diagnosis, they are free to leave my GP practice and seek alternative medicine.

Dr Philip: The patient certainly has this option but your role as a doctor is not to abandon your patient should your patient disagree with you. You should understand the patient, respect their beliefs, and try to help the patient understand that biomedicine adopts a different approach. In order to understand the patient, you first need to have acquired certain scientific knowledge from the social sciences.

Dr Philip opens his bag and takes out a book.

Dr Philip: This is the book we use for the sessions in sociology. It is titled *Applied Sociology of Health and Illness: A Problem-Based Learning Approach* (Second Edition) and it aims to apply sociological knowledge in order to understand real-life cases – cases that you may experience as clinicians in the future. In Chapter 1, for example, we learn about Alem Parkins who suffered a mild stroke, but she rejects any medical diagnoses. She attributes her experience to the evil eye inflicted on her by her British neighbour who she believes is jealous of her. Alem is a migrant from Ethiopia, where beliefs in the evil eye still prevail. Her doctor initially becomes frustrated and the two develop an awkward relationship. Alem does not trust modern medicine and her doctor is disappointed. However, her doctor receives advice from a colleague and attempts to recognise why Alem views the situation in the way she does and, thus, learns to respect her perception of her condition. In doing so, he eventually manages to help her decide that she needs to alter her lifestyle in order to benefit from improved health.

Frank: OK, I see the relevance in this case, but what about other situations? Earlier you mentioned something about the body as a 'social entity'. What do you mean by this?

Dr Philip: Could you look at the body of the student sitting to your left and tell me what social aspects relate to it?

> *Frank looks at the female student sitting to his left and with a puzzled expression on his face.*

Frank: Nothing!

Dr Philip: Well, as a sociologist, I see a woman who is wearing make-up, whose body is slim, who is dressed in jeans, like most of the other women in the audience.

Frank: How does this relate to sociology?

Dr Philip: Chapter 2 of the book explains that bodies become social because they carry the values of the societies they are in. Very often people are attracted to things that agree with the cultural values of respective societies. For example, a thin body is considered to be the ideal female figure among modern industrialised societies. People are socialised with such values from an early age, and they end up internalising or 'embodying' these values. As a result, people follow certain diets and engage in exercise or sport, eventually turning their bodies into 'projects' that are complete when the ideal body shape is achieved. 'Embodiment' and 'body project' are two of the concepts that Chapter 2 explores through the example of a young woman who cannot accept her body after she has gained weight due to her pregnancy. If you know that behind people's behaviour and preferences are certain cultural values, you can better understand them and help them find new ways to achieve their goals. For example, you may help them find other contexts of meaning such as being involved in social activities or groups.

Jessica (the student sitting next to Frank): Dr White, I like wearing make-up but I do not do it because my culture tells me to.

Dr Philip: Yes, of course. However, would you wear make-up if you grew up in a society that did not value make-up?

Frank: OK, I am starting to form a clearer picture now. You mentioned other areas in sociology, which you think are useful to us. For example, the way people experience a disease? I do not see any other way to experience a disease than to just seek treatment until a person is cured.

Dr Philip: Let us assume that you have a patient who suffers from kidney disease and is undergoing dialysis treatment while waiting for an organ for transplantation. You then find out that the patient is feeling depressed and anxious about the implications of haemodialysis. However, you do not really know why and need to talk to the patient in order to understand what is going on. Through talking with your patient, you learn about the patient's life, what they have achieved so far, how their life has changed because of the condition. This has been termed 'biographical disruption'. Such disruption might be devastating to a patient and, knowing how the patient experiences their condition, allows you to better comprehend the situation and, in turn, better communicate with them. In this way, you are able to help the patient to come to terms with their condition and to improve their level of adherence to the prescribed therapy. In this way, you avoid a situation whereby a patient may refuse to receive the dialysis treatment, which would lead to the deterioration of their condition, which ultimately would possibly become lethal. Chapter 3 discusses the main aspects of dealing with a chronic illness by focusing on the case of George Maros, who describes himself as a 'half-human'. By the end of the chapter, you come to understand that you need to learn about the patient, and not only about the part of their body that has malfunctioned. You are not just treating a body part; rather, you are treating a social human being. Additionally, patients may be labelled and stigmatised because of their health conditions.

Frank: What do you mean?

Dr Philip: How many of you know individuals who avoid socialising with other people, or going out to certain public places, as they fear standing out or being mocked on account of their condition?

Six students raise their hands.

Dr Philip: Yes, perhaps many more of you would raise your hands if you spent a little bit of time to consider the matter more carefully. What would you do if you had a patient who did not tell you important information about their condition because they felt ashamed? Under what circumstances would patients behave like that, do you think?

Frank: When they feel embarrassed about something?

Dr Philip: Exactly! If they feel embarrassed or stigmatised, they may be unable to express themselves or even go out and socialise with other people. This might happen in situations where other people know about one's condition or in cases where they do not. If they know, they may directly stigmatise the person by discriminating against them. On the other hand, if people are not aware of a person's condition, that person might hide their condition in order to avoid feeling stigmatised. These situations and types of stigmas are discussed in Chapter 4, which focuses on Mary Christian who does not want to visit public spaces; especially with her child as her child has Down syndrome. So, being aware of stigmatising circumstances, you may be able to help your patients deal with the issue and, thus, they may be more likely to confide in you and follow the recommended medication and therapy.

Frank: So, mental illness is a condition that is frequently stigmatised?

Dr Philip: Yes, Erving Goffman referred to this as 'blemishes of individual character', because it relates to people's behaviour. However, mental illness is not only socially managed but also socially influenced. In other words, social conditions or circumstances may contribute to the development of mental illnesses. If, for example, you knew a woman who was depressed, which factors would you attribute her depression to?

Frank: Upsetting circumstances in her life, loneliness perhaps.

Dr Philip: Yes, these might be possible reasons. You would understand much more if you knew that she was also a migrant, who was around 70 years old and living below the poverty line. Chapter 5 presents the relevant literature, which indicates that gender, migration, social class, and age are important factors that can affect the development of depression. However, you need to be careful. You should not take things for granted and make certain that you have a clear understanding of the patient's perspective.

Frank: What do you mean?

Dr Philip: In the scenario that appears in Chapter 5, Dr Jill Rogers makes a correct diagnosis that is based on the symptoms provided by the patient, Chun Bowie. However, Chun refuses to accept that she is suffering from depression and, consequently, she becomes angry and frustrated and leaves the hospital. What do you think about this situation?

Frank: Drawing from what you described to us about stigma, perhaps she feels that depression is a condition that stigmatises her?

Dr Philip: Yes, that might be a possibility. What other reasons can you identify?

Frank: Perhaps, it goes back to Chapter 1, which presents people's beliefs about health and illness. Perhaps Chun has her own theory about what is going on.

Dr Philip: Excellent, you are getting closer to the explanation! A medical student helps Dr Jill Rogers learn that depression, as a diagnosis, is not widely used in China, where Chun comes from. Instead, the term neurasthenia is used. This is because depression is considered to be socially and politically undesirable. So, people tend to express their feelings in physical, rather than psychological, terms and this is why neurasthenia is a more accepted term to use.

Frank: This is very interesting! Is this explained in Chapter 5?

Dr Philip: Yes. So, you see, Dr Jill Rogers might have approached her consultation differently had she had this information prior to her meeting with the patient.

Frank: Dr White, I understand that all this information is useful. However, you keep talking to us about individual cases. Are you sure that this relates to sociology and not psychology or communication studies?

Dr Philip: What makes you think that all this might be connected to psychology?

Frank: Well, sociology focuses on social groups and societies, not individuals.

Dr Philip: You are right to point out that sociology relates to social groups and societies. However, sociology also studies social behaviour or individuals as social beings in relation to other people. The individual cases, which I have already mentioned, serve as examples of wider trends that are present in societies. In other words, sociology can explain these individual cases and shed light on how we might handle them.

Frank: OK, that's good! Can you tell us what else we can learn from sociology?

Dr Philip: A classic question in the sociology of health is the following: do all people have the same life expectancy and do they get sick to the same extent? What do you think the answer to this might be?

Frank: I think that life expectancy and the likelihood of falling ill have to do with lifestyle and eating habits.

Dr Philip: That's true; anything else?

Jack: It could be related to where they live; in polluted areas, for example. Or it might be affected by the types of jobs that people perform?

Dr Philip: That's also true. Still, there are social factors or social characteristics that have a great influence on people's health. These are social class, gender, ethnicity, and age. Chapter 6 focuses on the relationship between social class and illness.

Frank: How can this be? Do you mean to say that working-class people, for example, have a lower life expectancy?

Dr Philip: Yes. The relationship between poverty and health was identified as early as the 19th century. Systematic research on the issue was conducted in the 1970s and 1980s and revealed that people from the lower social classes had higher mortality and morbidity rates. A famous study, conducted by Sir Douglas Black in the UK, resulted in publication of 'The Black Report', which discussed this relationship. Mr George Winters, the representative case in Chapter 6, is a man who resides below the poverty line. He has a heart attack but does not know that morbidity and mortality are linked to people's social status. When he finds out, he is disappointed and frustrated, but then realises that he cannot modify society or his financial position overnight. However, he is encouraged by his GP to change his lifestyle, by stopping or reducing his smoking and drinking habits, behaviours that are more likely to be observed among people from the lower social classes. His GP would not have been able to communicate this information to George and, eventually, help him to decide how to change his lifestyle if he did not know about the association between social class and lifestyle and illness.

I am sure that most of you have heard that women live longer than men, but they suffer from illnesses more than men. Is this indeed the case?

Melanie: Yes.

Dr Philip: Well, while it is true that women outlive men, the relevant literature does not seem to support the morbidity assumption. Women are more likely than men to have certain conditions, such as depression, but taking into account all medical conditions, there does not seem to be a difference. The discrepancy, however, lies with the reporting of illnesses. That is, women are more likely than men to report ill health. Chapter 7 discusses the reasons why this occurs. Women are seemingly more likely than men to consult a doctor at the initial stages of a medical condition, while men delay visiting a doctor until the symptoms worsen. Furthermore, health is associated with gender values and is connected to how men and women have been socialised in modern society. Chapter 7 does not focus on a specific health condition; rather, it presents the case of Graham Mayers who complains about the fact that women live longer than men. He is a heavy smoker and drinker who suffers from elevated blood pressure and cholesterol. Eventually, he is persuaded that certain health behaviours, such as smoking and alcohol abuse, are associated with manhood. With this in mind, it is much easier for him to try to change certain aspects of his lifestyle for the benefit of his good health.

Frank: This is very interesting. So women are not genetically predisposed or biologically protected (due to pregnancy) to live longer?

Dr Philip: Genetics and biological forces do play an important role. However, there are other reasons, such as: employment in dangerous jobs, lifestyle (men are more likely to be heavy smokers and drinkers), and risky activities (such as speeding). All these factors carry the values of power, autonomy, and independence, which societies consider as male values. Moreover, it is through these factors that men construct and maintain their masculine identity.

Society is a very powerful force in people's lives and health is not immune to it. To present another issue: what do you suppose is the relationship between ethnicity and health?

Michaela: Genetics.

Dr Philip: It could be. Anything else?

> *There is silence in the classroom. Nobody seems to have any other ideas.*

Dr Philip: Generally, migrants experience higher mortality and morbidity rates. There are many reasons for this, but the two most important are social class and racism. Migrants are more likely than native people to reside under the poverty line and, therefore, struggle with financial means. Also, they are prone to becoming victims of racism, or institutional racism, which may result in chronic stress and a deteriorated psychological state. These two social factors are analysed in Chapter 8, where the case of Anup Banerjee, a Bangladeshi migrant in the UK, is presented. As clinicians, you should do your best to ensure that migrant patients do not experience any institutional racism through your practice. Moreover, you could provide them with some sound advice as to how they might increase their social support networks.

Frank: Dr White, you have not mentioned anything about age and health. We live in an ageing society and knowing the social and medical implications would be very useful.

Dr Philip: How would it be useful to you?

Frank: I remember reading a related article the other day, which stressed that older people are likely to have chronic conditions. This means that people nowadays live longer than ever before, but they are not well. Also, older people may find themselves isolated, without any networks that could provide them with social support. Alternatively, older people might find that they need care from other people who are close to them, such as their children or grandchildren.

Dr Philip: In sociology, this is called 'informal care', and the matter is discussed in Chapter 9 along with other issues you have raised. The chapter describes the experiences of David Gordon, who is 80 years old, suffers from a chronic condition, yet he does not feel old. As the chapter progresses, his condition deteriorates, which leaves him incapable of taking care of himself and, as a result, he requires an informal carer for his daily needs and survival. The informal carer in this case is his wife.

Frank: Does he die, eventually?

Dr Philip: He does, and Chapter 9 also presents the social aspects of dying and death. That is, in the chapter you will learn about social death, as compared to biological death; how death used to be part of daily life but, over time, it became medically interesting – what sociologists call the 'medicalisation of death' – and how death has now become a part of the medical intervention provided by hospitals. As future clinicians, you will be faced with dying patients and their relatives and loved ones. Your role does not necessarily end where medicine does.

Frank: What do you mean?

Dr Philip: Would you inform the patient or the relatives about the imminent death?

Frank: I am not sure.

Natalie: I don't think that I would; the patient would give up their struggle to live sooner and patients need to have hope.

Jessica: I would; if a patient is dying, they have the right to know.

Kevin: I agree. If a patient knows that they are dying, certain actions might be taken to prepare. For example, saying goodbye, making amends, connecting with friends or relatives that they have not had the chance to see for a long time, and so on.

Dr Philip: Sociologically speaking, you have touched on the issue of 'closed' and 'open' awareness. Open awareness is most common in the West, nowadays, and it has been associated with the term 'good death'. Death is defined as good because the dying person has the chance to resolve any pending issues and say goodbye to friends and relatives. As clinicians, you will be faced with the dilemma of closed or open awareness, depending on the case, but you will possibly need to abide by your hospitals' policy regarding the matter.

Frank: All of the topics that you have presented seem very interesting. You have also mentioned 'digital health'. I am not familiar with this term

Dr Philip: Digital health is a recent concept which captures the development of technologies (e.g., apps, smart watches, etc.) to help patients monitor their health. In the last chapter of the book students learn about John Goodman who is 60 years old and has prediabetes. Because of his very busy schedule he expresses concerns about his capacity to monitor his glucose levels, diet, and exercise and his doctor advises to check any digital options which can help him. Although John finds a few options which could potentially help him he learns that he has to be careful with the type of technology he uses and discusses the issue with his doctor. He also learns that digital health technologies are not for everybody in the sense that access is limited by socioeconomic background and education.

Frank: That's also interesting. Are we going to go over all these topics during our lectures?

Dr Philip: Yes, and we will use this book as a guide. It functions as a guide for two reasons. *First,* it draws from the relevant literature to inform real-life cases. In other words, it works like problem-based learning (PBL) or cased-based learning (CBL) cases that you have in your curriculum, but here we are using sociological knowledge to make sense of them. You can use the book individually and follow the instructions. That is, you read the scenario, think of the questions in boxes, go through the literature, and then explain the scenario. This can also be done in small groups. *Second,* the book does not exhaust the literature; it merely covers the basic theories and serves as a starting point. Should you need to develop a deeper understanding of the subject, you should explore the issues using other textbooks or academic articles.

Frank: Though I initially challenged the usefulness of sociology, I must admit that it seems to be necessary for all health professionals. I still need to learn more and attend the lectures in order to realise just how useful it is. Where can we find the book?

Dr Philip: That's alright! I understand your initial reluctance; you are not the only student who raised concerns. You could attend all the sociology lectures and borrow the book from the library to begin with. I wish you all the best and should you have any questions about sociology, please feel free to contact me. Carol, I am sorry for taking up so much of your time, but I think it was useful for the students.

Professor Carol: That's perfectly alright; I had finished my slides anyway. It was very helpful, Philip. I think we should organise similar sessions for all the social sciences so that students have the opportunity to pose questions and reflect on the material they will be taught.

Professor Carol: Thank you for your attendance, and I wish you all the best on your new journey as medical students.

Frank Bennet is now more interested in the subject and visits the library in order to borrow the book that Dr Philip White had used to explain how sociology could be useful to healthcare students and practitioners. He looks forward to the first sociology session, which is scheduled to take place next week and he hopes that he will not be disappointed. He opens the book to the first chapter and begins to read about the case of Alem Parkins. He recalls from Dr Philip White's presentation that this is the patient who believes that her stroke was caused as a result of her neighbour inflicting the 'evil eye' on her. Frank continues reading through the chapter.

CHAPTER 1

Lay health beliefs and doctor–patient relationships

....

ABSTRACT

Mrs Alem Parkins suffered a mild stroke and was brought to the emergency unit at a local hospital. However, she refuses to accept any of the medical diagnoses provided by the doctors and develops her own conclusions as to what happened to her. Relevant literature indicates that laypersons, like Alem, rely on many sources such as modern biomedicine, cultural and religious values, and personal experiences to develop their own theories and beliefs about health and the causes of diseases. This chapter illustrates how sociological information could assist healthcare students and practitioners in better understanding why a patient, such as Alem, may have specific health beliefs. It also presents how healthcare students and practitioners should approach and treat a patient whose health beliefs are far different from Western biomedical philosophy.

LEARNING OBJECTIVES

- Explain what the term lay health beliefs means.
- Identify and describe specific lay health beliefs.
- Distinguish and explain the difference between cultural and scientific approaches to health and illness causation.

DOI: 10.1201/9781003256687-2

- Discern the main types of doctor–patient relationships.
- Outline cultural competence and its importance.

Note: Think about or discuss the questions that are in the boxes before you continue reading through the chapter.

SCENARIO

Mrs Alem Parkins is rushed to the hospital by her son after she fainted while shopping at a popular shopping mall. Her son initially thought that his mother had collapsed due to the fatigue she had been experiencing over the past few days. At the emergency unit, he told the doctor, 'She has been overworked and she collapsed'. Fortunately, the doctor saw that Mrs Parkins was breathing but he could hardly find her pulse. She was immediately given oxygen and a medical team started examining her thoroughly. The medical diagnosis was that she had suffered a mild stroke. Mrs Parkins woke up the next day and was informed of her condition. However, she could not accept that she had suffered a stroke.

DISCUSS

1. Why does Alem Parkins not accept the medical diagnosis as valid?
2. Is it possible that Alem will ask for a second diagnosis at a different hospital? .
3. What could her explanation be, concerning what happened to her?

FURTHER DEVELOPMENTS

Dr Eric Johnson: Good morning, Mrs Parkins. How do you feel today?
Alem: Exhausted. I feel like I fell off a skyscraper!
Dr Eric: It is normal to feel this way after what you have experienced.
Alem: What happened, Doctor?
Dr Eric: You had a mild stroke, which does not seem to have left any serious consequences.
Alem: A stroke? What's that?
Dr Eric: Well, a stroke is also called a brain attack and happens when blood stops flowing to some areas in your brain.

Alem: And why does it stop? [*Alem's facial expressions cause Dr Eric to start feeling somewhat uncomfortable.*]

Dr Eric: The risk factors are numerous. For example, diabetes, ageing, high cholesterol, high blood pressure, and so on. It seems that yours might have been due to chronic high blood pressure.

Alem: And how do you know that?

Dr Eric: High blood pressure is one of the main risk factors, and your medical history records show that you have had chronic high blood pressure, which was not managed by medication.

Alem: And based on a piece of paper you conclude that high blood pressure is the cause?

Dr Eric: The examination has showed that your brain arteries have been damaged, possibly due to chronic high blood pressure.

> *Falling silent suddenly, Alem looks at the floor and takes a deep breath. She then turns to Dr Eric Johnson and says harshly:*

> Doctor, I believe that you don't really know what is wrong with me. You just can't know what is going on inside my body. It is my body, not yours! I know much better than you what is happening inside my body and what made me collapse. It is the evil eye that other people have brought upon my body. My condition has nothing to do with a stroke or my arteries! I am not sick. I feel fine. I am just a little tired.

> *Dr Eric Johnson does not respond; he feels quite upset and is ready to tell Alem off. He manages to control himself and leaves the room without saying a word.*

DISCUSS

1. Why does Alem refuse to accept that she has suffered a stroke?
2. What does she mean by saying that the evil eye is the main cause of her collapse?
3. How can you better understand her belief in the evil eye.
4. What does she mean when she says that she is not sick but, rather, simply tired?
5. Why did Dr Eric Johnson become upset and leave the room without talking to Mrs Parkins?

FURTHER DEVELOPMENTS

Dr Eric Johnson is angry and asks his colleague, Dr Petra Miles, to drop by his office for support. Dr Miles explains that patients come to the doctor with their own beliefs and that this is not the first time they have experienced this. She encourages Dr Johnson to accept the situation, reapproach the patient, and give her space to explain her perspective.

DISCUSS

1. How do patients come up with their own diagnoses and theories about health?
2. What sources do laypeople and doctors utilise in order to understand health and illness?
3. What further information do you need to answer these questions?

A VERY BRIEF HISTORY OF LAY PERCEPTIONS OF DISEASES

Dr Petra Miles is correct to note that people develop their own theories of what causes a disease and what health is (Nettleton, 2006). However, people do not develop beliefs about health and illness randomly. Instead, they draw information from their rich cognitive template, which has largely been shaped by cultural and religious values, social relations experienced throughout their lives, and the threatening diseases to which they risked exposure. In medieval times, for example, people believed that epidemics and deadly diseases were a form of punishment inflicted by God on people whose behaviour deviated from the moral norm (Adam and Herzlich, 1994). Over the centuries, the diseases that killed thousands of people in medieval times were controlled, largely due to the improvement of living conditions, which resulted in an increase in the life expectancy and size of the population – a phenomenon that has been termed 'demographic transition' (Bury, 1997, p. 9) (see Chapter 9, 'Ageing Society and Older People', for more information about demographic transition).

Modern biomedicine and the introduction of vaccinations in the early 20th century have further contributed to controlling diseases that used to be terminal. Such developments have had an impact on people's understandings of health and expanded their template to attribute diseases to factors other than God, such as the environment and lifestyle (Helman, 2007). Diseases in the 20th and 21st centuries are different from diseases experienced in the past. Modern medical conditions, such as coronary diseases, degenerative diseases, stroke, and cancer, are chronic and some conditions may be associated with lifestyle. Going through these sociohistorical changes has caused people in modern times to draw from a variety of sources so as to better understand health and illness and seek medical help (Taber, Leyva, and Persoskie, 2015). They may rely on modern biomedicine, cultural and religious values, and personal experience to formulate their attitudes and beliefs of what health is and what causes diseases.

The availability of complementary and alternative medicine (CAM) has also contributed to how people understand and appreciate conventional treatment. CAM includes therapies which do not fall under the conventional biomedical ways of treatment, such as, for example, acupuncture, homeopathy, and chiropractics, which have been popular in the recent times (Frass et al., 2012). Interestingly, earlier studies showed that the use of CAM was influenced by social characteristics, such as gender and socioeconomic background (Astin, 1998; Kelner and Wellman, 1997). In support, Fjaer et al. (2020) conducted a pan-European study, collecting data from 21 countries and 33,371 participants, in order to illuminate the social reasons why people are increasingly using CAM therapies and identify any differences across countries. They concluded that women, people with higher socioeconomic status, with higher education, people who had unmet healthcare needs, and those who were not satisfied with conventional therapies were more likely to use CAM. Any differences between countries were related to each country's expenditure, resulting in the availability of more or fewer CAM options for people.

DISCUSS

1. Based on the information above, how would you explain Alem's behaviour?
2. What other information do you need from the relevant literature in order to further understand Alem's behaviour?

BELIEFS ABOUT ILLNESS CAUSATION AND HEALTH

Alem lives in London. However, she was born and raised in the Amhara area of Ethiopia where belief in the evil eye still prevails. She has been socialised with such beliefs and has learned that illness and misfortune can be attributed to the act of the evil eye, which can be inflicted by other people who are jealous and may wish to cause her harm. She moved to the United Kingdom when she was 20 years old and has lived there since. She is now 42 years old. Alem has experiences from two different cultures. However, she does not seem to have embraced modern biomedicine as practised in London. Her behaviour highlights two main areas that require special attention: (1) understanding illness causation and (2) beliefs about health.

Understanding illness causation

Alem's understanding of the causation of illness accords with Helman's (2007, p. 134) approach, which presents 'the social world' as one of the sites where people locate the causes of diseases. Helman outlines witchcraft, sorcery, and the evil eye as examples of illness causation in this site. These are believed to be inflicted by some people in various communities around the globe due to jealousy and conflict. Helman refers to three more sites where laypeople place the causes of disease. These are 'the individual world', 'the natural world', and 'the supernatural world'. Locating the causes of a disease within the individual world means that the disease manifests itself in malfunctioning organs and this may be attributed to individual behaviour, such as food consumption. The natural world may be understood as an important site outside the individual, where environmental factors, such as cold, heat, and humidity, may have an impact on people's health. In the supernatural world, it is believed that various supernatural entities, such as gods and spirits, observe people on Earth and may inflict diseases as a form of punishment should the living people violate fundamental social rules or do not honour these supernatural entities properly.

Other scholars would have classified Alem's understanding of the causation of her illness under different categories. For example, Singer and Baer (2007, p. 70) outlined four theories of illness. These are: theories of 'natural causation' (e.g., infection, accident), 'supernatural causation' (e.g., fate, contagion), 'animistic causation' (e.g., spirit aggression), and 'magical causation' (e.g., sorcery and witchcraft). On the basis of these theories, Alem employs the theory of magical causation.

Helman clarifies that the social and the supernatural worlds, as sites for a disease, are largely observed in non-Western countries, whereas in Western societies, the sites of the individual and the natural world tend to dominate. In support, Waskul and Eaton (2018) explained that attributing the causes of illness to the social and supernatural worlds is more prominent in non-Western countries or among migrants from African and Asian countries residing in the West. However, attributing illness to the social world has been observed in the Western world as well. For example, Waskul and Eaton (2018) explained that recent surveys among university students in the United States indicated that belief in supernatural entities was quite common. Along similar lines, Roussou (2014) argued that belief in the evil eye was not unique to non-Western countries and that it is still prevalent in modern Greece.

Beliefs about health

Apart from the social world to which Alem attributes the cause of her stroke, her words also reveal how she views and understands health in general. While talking with Dr Johnson, she explains that she is not sick and that what she really needs is some rest so that she can go back to her usual routine. Alem's belief about health is an example of what Blaxter (2010, p. 8) termed 'health as function', a phrase used to explain that people understand health as the ability to act in two different ways. *First*, health equals the ability to do things in daily life and to be engaged in social activities. As Blaxter (2010, p. 9) put it, 'disease is failure in adaptation, and is dysfunctional both to individuals themselves and to the societies of which they are part'. *Second*, health is the ability to achieve personal and cultural goals. In other words, if people do not identify any physical changes, which may lead to discomfort, and can still fulfil social obligations and complete daily tasks, they then identify themselves as healthy.

Alem's beliefs coincide with findings from other scholars. For example, an early work in France by Herzlich (1973) showed that laypeople understood that individuals were innately healthy, and that disease existed as a possible threat. People tended to view themselves as healthy when they could not identify any symptoms and understand that disease comes from the physical and social environment. Herzlich (1973, p. 63) went on to identify three main perceptions of health: 'health in a vacuum', 'reserve of health', and 'health as equilibrium'. Health in a vacuum refers to perceptions of a healthy individual when no disease has been identified or has developed. Reserve of health has more to do with the individual's capacities, such as how strong their body is to resist diseases and the individual's ability to cope with daily stress. Finally, health as equilibrium refers to maintaining the balance inside the body and between the individual and the social world.

Hughner and Kleine (2004) reviewed the literature of the studies of lay health beliefs and outlined 18 lay understandings of health, which seem to support the findings of both Herzlich and Blaxter. These lay understandings of health can be divided into two main domains: intrinsic and extrinsic. The intrinsic domain refers to beliefs in the role of natural factors such as genetics, the function of organs, and so forth; for example, a woman who is believed to have developed breast cancer due to a genetic predisposition. The extrinsic domain relates to beliefs in individual acts, social relations, and the environment. For example, work conditions, individual responsibility, and lifestyle (e.g., smoking) are examples of the extrinsic factors that influence health.

A review of the literature related to the health beliefs of women in the United States who were born in Asia showed interesting findings (Zhao et al., 2010). Vietnamese women defined health as the absence of a disease by arguing that there was no cancer if there were no symptoms. Korean women viewed cancer as a form of punishment by God, but they also placed particular emphasis on lifestyle by arguing that diet and stress have an impact on health. They recommended faith in God as a way to maintain health (along similar lines, Rothstein and Rajapaksa (2003) found that Indians valued religious faith as an important factor for being healthy). Zhao et al. (2010) went on to explain that Hmong people understood health as the absence of a medical condition; however, they also focused on the importance of family equilibrium in achieving a healthy life. Interestingly, Chinese participants stressed the importance of maintaining a good balance in one's life, social relations, and food consumption (see also Lai and Surood, 2009). Kilby and Sherman (2018) clarified that lay beliefs about health and healthcare are dynamic and are constantly informed by many sources, including scientific information.

Returning to the case of Alem, she believes in the act of the evil eye and, as such, does not embrace modern biomedicine's approach to her health condition. She does not believe that she is sick and that she could not keep up with her normal routine. It also appears that she and her doctor are in conflict with one another. Let us now see how the story will develop given that Dr Johnson does not seem to accept Alem's stance as rational.

FURTHER DEVELOPMENTS

Dr Johnson returns to Alem to explain more about her condition and to clarify the medical point of view that led to the diagnosis. He finds his patient talking on her cell phone and overhears

Alem making plans to meet with her friends later on. When Alem notices that the doctor has entered the room, she ends her telephone call in order to speak with him.

Dr Eric: Mrs Parkins, you have to get some rest and take your medication regularly. Also, the nurse will give you some useful information about following a recommended diet in order to maintain normal blood pressure and reduce the risks of having another stroke.

Alem: Thank you, Doctor. However, I plan on reducing the risk of having another stroke by taking the proper precautions. I think that my British neighbour envies my relaxed way of life and therefore gave me the evil eye. I may need to visit a specialist that can cast out the evil eye.

Dr Eric: Mrs Parkins, I insist that you have to be very careful with your blood pressure. We are here to help you with any questions you may have.

DISCUSS

1. What kind of a relationship has developed between Alem and Dr Johnson?
2. Why is there a big difference between lay and scientific knowledge?
3. What sources do laypeople and doctors utilise in order to understand health and illness?

THE LAY AND SCIENTIFIC KNOWLEDGE, AND DOCTOR–PATIENT RELATIONSHIPS

It is certain that Alem and Dr Eric Johnson cannot communicate effectively, and they have trouble listening to one another, while Dr Johnson seems to be adopting a more paternalistic relationship (Silverman, Kurtz, and Draper, 2016). The scene described above highlights two important issues that deserve further examination. The *first* issue has to do with the different philosophies Alem and Dr Johnson rely on in order to understand health. The *second* relates to the relationship between Alem and her doctor. Let me now discuss further Alem and Dr Johnson's different philosophies.

Dr Johnson has been trained as a doctor in modern medicine, which adopts the biomedical model for understanding and curing a disease. The biomedical model relies heavily on scientific knowledge, separates mind from body and focuses on the latter, understands diseases as entities that can be identified, measured, and controlled, and places particular emphasis on the individual rather than the social world (Helman, 2007). In other words, modern medicine aims at an objective measurement (through identifiable symptoms, which are distinct across diseases) and management (cure of a disease or control over the symptoms) of physical changes inside the human body (Nettleton, 2006). In addition, modern medicine focuses, with the help of epidemiology, on individual behaviour, such as diet and lifestyle, in order to explain or predict the development of certain diseases (e.g., heart diseases or some types of cancer). This has turned modern medicine into a system of social control, which dictates to people specific ways in which to live their lives (Zola, 1972). 'Cultural iatrogenesis' is a term that has been used to describe the process of controlling people's lives through modern medicine (Illich, 1976, p. 42). Cultural iatrogenesis derives from the medicalisation of a person's life, which refers to the increasing number of aspects of a person's life that are put under medical scrutiny and intervention (Zola, 1972). Medicalisation is further analysed in Chapter 2, 'The Body as a Social Entity'.

Alem, on the other hand, relies heavily on cultural knowledge concerning the cause and treatment of a disease and, more specifically, on her belief in the evil eye. Beliefs in the evil eye have been observed in many areas of the world, such as Greece, Italy, Turkey, Iran, and the Middle East (Helman, 2007). In Greece, for example, Herzfeld (1981) asserted that the evil eye was a condition that was inherent in social relations and was used as a way to make sense of misfortunes and individual misconduct (see also Roussou, 2014). People who have been socially marginalised, are childless, and those who are jealous by nature are likely to be considered as possessors of the evil eye. On the basis of these attributes, older women, according to Herzfeld (1981), were very often ascribed such qualities. Along similar lines, Galt (1982) stressed that one of the main attributes of the evil eye on the island of Pantelleria in Italy was jealousy.

The evil eye in the area of Amhara in Ethiopia, where Alem is from, has been studied by Reminick (1974). Reminick (1974, p. 280) found that the people who had the power of the evil eye, the 'buda' (see also Baynes-Rock, 2015), were not the Amhara people but people from other areas. Someone who was good looking or had beautiful children was more susceptible to a buda attack. The way out of the evil eye was a ritualistic attack on it, usually by a specialist. These cultural beliefs have shaped people's way of thinking about misfortune, which Alem still carries in her cognitive template. They were deeply ingrained in Alem's social and cognitive map and became second nature or what Bourdieu (1991, p. 12) has called 'habitus', which refers to 'a set of dispositions which incline agents to act and react in certain ways'.

The second issue that deserves close attention is the relationship that has developed between Alem and her doctor. Doctors and patients are two different social agents who are likely to have different cultural and religious backgrounds and knowledge about health and illness. They may also enjoy different social statuses, especially if the patient hails from a working-class background. The relationship between the two is a power relationship in the sense that the doctor possesses the knowledge to understand and cure a disease and the patient relies exclusively on the doctor for dealing with a health condition. Doctors gained their power to practise in many Western countries during the last 100 years when guidelines and regulations were enacted to legitimate the physician's profession, and new medical discoveries cured many infectious diseases (Fitzpatrick and Speed, 2018; Adam and Herzlich, 1994; Scambler, 2008).

However, without authority doctors cannot diagnose and treat patients. They need authority in order to inform patients about health conditions, to help patients decide what is the best treatment for them, and to treat and communicate effectively with patients (Silverman, Kurtz, and Draper, 2016). Within this context, specific types of relationships develop between doctors and patients. Early theory on doctor–patient relationships was developed by Szasz and Hollender (1956) that outlined three types of relationships. *First*, in cases where the patient cannot respond, the patient is a de facto passive recipient of medical treatment. *Second*, in cases in which the patient can communicate, the patient listens and agrees with the doctor's assessments. *Third*, both the doctor and the patients may collaborate in the assessment and management of the disease.

Dr Johnson is trying to develop a relationship in which Alem adheres to her doctor's advice. There are no signs of collaboration in the communication between the two and, perhaps, this is one of the reasons Alem cannot trust her doctor. The relationship that is developing between the two is that of conflict, which echoes Freidson (1970) who explained that both doctors and patients are likely to deviate from their social roles and may come into conflict due to the different social and cultural backgrounds they have, as well as the distinct knowledge about health and illness which they possess.

Such a relationship of conflict puts in jeopardy the social roles that both Alem and Dr Johnson are expected to perform and, as a result, challenges the approach of Parsons (1952) who explained that once a person becomes sick, both the doctor and the patient have to perform specific roles in order to achieve the best outcome – that is, to cure the patient (see Chapter 3 for more information about the 'sick role'). On the one hand, the doctor is expected to apply their medical knowledge to understand and cure the condition by putting any biases against the patient aside. On the other hand, the patient is absolved of blame for their medical condition and is expected to withdraw from social activities, seek medical help, and adhere to medical treatment in order to be well and return to the social world. Thereafter, the doctor and the patient need to collaborate on the basis of their own different roles in order to achieve an effective consultation and the best possible outcome. Echoing Parsons, Silverman, Kurtz, and Draper (2016) explained that one of the fundamental parts of a medical consultation is to listen to the patient carefully and give them the opportunity to present their situation. Alem's case seems to deviate from this procedure because she has not been motivated to tell her doctors more about her condition; what she has said about the evil eye has not been accepted by her doctor and she does not seem to be willing to adhere to any medical treatment.

Although consultation has turned from doctor-centred to patient-centred in recent decades (Silverman, Kurtz, and Draper, 2016; May et al., 2004), Dr Johnson adopts a doctor-centred approach by regarding Alem's stance as illegitimate and by presenting his decision as what Alem has to accept. Dr Johnson's behaviour resonates with the research findings by Braddock et al. (1997), who analysed 88 patient visits to physicians. The authors found that physicians focused on explaining the medical condition; they tended not to outline any risks or benefits and were inclined not to place any emphasis on patients' comprehension of what course of medical treatment had been decided. Moreover, there is no sign of empathy in Dr Johnson's dialogue, and this is a factor that contributes to maintaining his conflict with Alem. Chipidza, Wallwork, and Stern (2015) stressed that good doctor–patient relationships may fail to develop when there is a lack of trust, and when doctors do not take the time to explain their reasoning adequately and do not establish a good rapport with their patients. On this note, Dr Johnson ought to follow a different approach in order to observe a change in Alem's behaviour.

The relationship between Dr Johnson and Alem shows the existence of two different regimes of knowledge, namely medicine and lay understanding. Nowadays, doctors learn how to practise patient-centred care, despite medicine's dominance in modern society. It is interesting to discuss briefly how medicine has come to dominate healthcare.

Medicine did not have a dominant position in society before the 19th century, when doctors were a minority among other healthcare providers, such as homeopathic healers and midwives (Scambler, 2008). Doctors at the time were trained only in the basic functions of the body; they were not initially trained in hospitals, which were not considered safe places for patients (Fitzpatrick and Speed, 2018; Morgan, 2008).

Modern medicine developed as a professional discipline in the 19th century, and it developed alongside advances in science (Crinson, 2008; Morgan, 2008). The 19th century was the time when medicine in the United States, for example, was increasingly offered at universities, and professional standards were introduced, so by the end of the century a licence was necessary to practise medicine. Advances in science, such as the use of anaesthesia, antiseptic, surgery, etc., further pushed medicine as a profession that would help humanity thrive (Fitzpatrick and Speed, 2018). Medical successes in dealing with health issues at the time helped gain public respect. That is, the development of vaccines which cured infectious diseases in early 20th century and the epidemiology and statistics which provided insights into the distribution of diseases in the population and potential risk factors for serious diseases, provided solid ground for instilling medicine's position in modern society. In addition, political and historical circumstances indicated that medicine was needed more than ever before. Specifically, civil war in the United States in the 19th century and the two world wars in the 20th century revealed the urgent need to improve and expand medical treatment and hospitalisation, and to enhance medical education. Moreover, scientific medicine evolved and many medical associations as well as scientific journals emerged in the context of nurturing evidence-based medicine and guiding policies and directions regarding people's healthy lifestyle. In the 20th century, organisations such as the World Health Organization (WHO), were established, aiming to improve global health (see Chapter 6). The recent COVID-19 pandemic shows that nowadays medicine is the dominant regime of knowledge for informing decisions about public health, confirming that it has a well-established position in the modern era (see Chapter 6).

Despite the development of modern medicine in Western industrialised countries, it has its limitations, such as the medicalisation of aspects of life which were not under medical scrutiny before, like for instance homosexuality, childbirth, and obesity. Homosexuality was considered a pathology and was medically treated until the early 1970s, which resulted in the stigmatisation and isolation of people who disclosed their homosexual orientation. Medicalisation of childbirth contributed towards improved survival rates for both infants and their mothers but put women under the scrutiny of science, undermining their decisions regarding where and how to give birth. Although, medicalisation of obesity is still debated today (see Chapter 2), it resulted in pathologising lifestyle and stigmatising obese people, even if they were healthy (Wilding, Mooney, and Pile, 2019). Criticism of modern medicine for having medicalised normal aspects of life has contributed towards a more patient-centred care, which began taking form between 1950 and 1980 (Armstrong, 2011) and was more widely practised and introduced in medical practice in the 1980s (Morgan, 2008).

DISCUSS

1. Having this knowledge, how should Dr Johnson approach the patient?
2. Which concepts and guidelines in the literature can help you answer this question?

FURTHER DEVELOPMENTS

Dr Johnson starts feeling frustrated again and wants to leave the room. He feels that he cannot handle the situation and considers calling Dr Miles for further assistance. Before leaving the room, however, Alem responds to Dr Johnson's advice about her blood pressure.

Alem: Don't worry; my blood pressure will be under control as soon as I remove the evil eye from my body.

Dr Eric picks up the opportunity and changes direction, remembering Dr Miles's advice about giving the patient space to explain her perspective.

Dr Eric: How does this work?
Alem: Once the evil eye is out, I will be more relaxed and careful with my lifestyle.
Dr Eric: What do you mean? Please tell me more.
Alem: If I am free of it, I can then be more cautious with my life.
Dr Eric: So you think that the evil eye prevents you from leading a healthier life?
Alem: That's for sure. It will not let me open my eyes and see the dangers.

Dr Eric: I understand that the evil eye is a problem for you. You can do whatever you need to do to remove it, provided it does not cause any harm. I would be happy if you informed me when it is out, and you have started leading a healthier life. I was not aware of these issues. You know, at my medical school we did not learn about cultural understandings of health and diseases but only about scientific measurements and the identification and classification of symptoms. Symptoms result from physical changes due to diseases. This is how we, doctors, understand a person's body and health and this is why I focused on the damage that your chronic blood pressure has left on your arteries. It is interesting that I now know your explanation.

Alem: I am glad; it is a good thing that you do not think I am crazy and that you did not refer me to a psychiatrist! Getting rid of the evil eye requires a specialist that will use prayer for the matter.

Dr Eric [smiles]: Don't worry about it, Mrs Parkins. Now that you have two diagnoses, perhaps it would be a good idea to get rid of the evil eye, take your medication and be more careful with your lifestyle.

Alem: Yes, this is a good plan. I just need to get out of here as soon as possible in order to meet with a friend who can help me to cast out the evil eye.

DISCUSS

1. Does the above conversation bring about any changes in the relationship between Alem and Dr Johnson?
2. Is there anything new in how Alem understands health and the causes of diseases?

DOCTOR–PATIENT RELATIONSHIPS AND CULTURAL COMPETENCE

Interestingly, a turn in the relationship between Alem and Dr Johnson is observed. Dr Johnson does not reject Alem's understanding of what caused her stroke. He is not judgemental, shows respect and, more importantly, he demonstrates a genuine interest in learning more about her beliefs. His behaviour shows that he now values Alem's perception and beliefs and, as a result, he manages to build trust between the two of them. Alem feels closer to Dr Johnson, who appears to be more accepting of her views. Thus, she is keener to accept his advice on medication and lifestyle. This shows the importance of listening to and understanding patients (Silverman, Kurtz, and Draper, 2016). Alem and Dr Johnson have negotiated and learned from each other. Their approaches to the causes of the illness are still in conflict with one another, but they have managed to agree on the course of treatment. Dr Johnson is establishing a more mutual relationship, whereby the doctor and the patient are on the same page and decide together (Silverman, Kurtz, and Draper, 2016). Dr Johnson's approach reflects cultural competence (Constantinou et al., 2018; Constantinou et al., 2020), which refers to an understanding of social and cultural factors which influence illness and the management of conditions, and actions or interventions aiming to provide the best possible care to patients regardless of their background (Betancourt, 2003). There are other concepts which fall under the umbrella of cultural competence or have been used as additional or clearer captures of what it means to work with diversity, such as intercultural competence, cultural humility, structured competence, and so forth. Studies show that cultural competence has been associated with patient satisfaction and adherence to therapy (Horvat et al., 2014; Renzaho et al., 2013; Beach et al., 2005). In Alem's case, a culturally competent doctor helped her feel listened to and understood, and she started embracing biomedical advice for improving her condition. Cultural and diversity competence skills relate to all the chapters of this book.

FURTHER DEVELOPMENTS

Having established a good relationship with Alem Parkins, Dr Johnson calls for a medical staff meeting to share his experience and discuss the issue of training all medical professionals at the hospital in the basic sociological principles of lay health beliefs and their implications, in cultural competence, and in how to build effective relationships with patients through improving communication skills.

REFERENCES

Adam P, Herzlich C. *Sociologie de la Maladie et de la Médicine.* Paris: Nathan; 1994.

Armstrong D. The invention of patient-centred medicine. *Soc Theory Health.* 2011; 9(4): 410–8.

Astin JA. Why patients use alternative medicine: Results of a national study. *JAMA.* 1998; 279(19): 1548–53.

Baynes-Rock M. Ethiopian buda as hyenas: Where the social is more than human. *Folklore.* 2015; 126(3): 266–82.

Beach MC, Price EG, Gary TL, Robinson KA, Gozu A, Palacio A, Smarth C, Jenckes M, Feuerstein C, Bass EB, Powe NR. A systematic review of the methodological rigor of studies evaluating cultural competence training of health professionals. *Acad Med.* 2005; 80(6): 578–86.

Betancourt J, Green AR, Carrillo JE, Ananeh-Firempong O. Defining cultural competence: A practical framework for addressing racial / ethnic disparities in health and health care. *Public Health Rep.* 2003; 118: 293–302.

Blaxter M. *Health.* 2nd ed. Cambridge: Polity Press; 2010.

Bourdieu P. *Language and Symbolic Power.* Cambridge, MA: Harvard University Press; 1991.

Braddock CH, Fihn SD, Levinson W, Jonsen AR, Pearlman RA. How doctors and patients discuss routine clinical decisions: Informed decision making in the outpatient setting. *J Gen Int Med.* 1997; 12(6): 339–45.

Bury M. *Health and Illness in a Changing Society.* New York: Routledge; 1997.

Chipidza FE, Wallwork RS, Stern TA. Impact of the doctor-patient relationship. *Prim Care Companion CNS Disord.* 2015; 17(5). 10.4088/PCC.15f01840.

Constantinou CS, Andreou P, Papageorgiou A, McCrorie P. Critical reflection on own beliefs for cultural competence in medical education: An analysis of tutors' reflective narratives. *Qual Res Educ.* 2020; 9(3): 273–99.

Constantinou CS, Papageorgiou A, Samoutis G, McCrorie P. Acquire, apply, and activate knowledge: A pyramid model for teaching and integrating cultural competence in medical curricula. *Patient Educ Couns.* 2018; 101(6): 1147–51.

Crinson I. The health professions. In: Scambler G, editor. *Sociology as Applied to Medicine*, pp. 252–264. London: Elsevier Health Sciences; 2008.

Fitzpatrick R, Speed E. Society and changing patterns of health and illness. In: Scambler G, editor. *Sociology as Applied to Medicine*, pp. 3–17. 7th ed. London: Palgrave; 2018.

Fjær EL, Landet ER, McNamara CL, Eikemo TA. The use of complementary and alternative medicine (CAM) in Europe. *BMC Complement. Med. Therapies* 2020; 20(1): 1–9.

Frass M, Strassl RP, Friehs H, Müllner M, Kundi M, Kaye AD. Use and acceptance of complementary and alternative medicine among the general population and medical personnel: a systematic review. *Ochsner J.* 2012; 12(1): 45–56.

Friedson E. *Profession of Medicine: A Study of the Sociology of Applied Knowledge.* Chicago, IL: University of Chicago Press; 1970.

Galt AH. The evil eye as synthetic image and its meanings on the island of Pantelleria, Italy. *Am Ethnol.* 1982; 9(4): 664–81.

Helman CG. *Culture, Health and Illness.* 5th ed. London: Hodder Education; 2007.

Herzfeld M. Meaning and morality: A semiotic approach to evil eye accusations in a Greek village. *American Ethnol.* 1981; 8(3): 560–74.

Herzlich C. *Health and Illness: A Social Psychological Analysis.* London: European Association of Experimental Social Psychology, Academic Press; 1973.

Horvat L, Horey D, Romios P, Kis-Rigo J. Cultural competence education for health professionals. *Cochrane Database Syst Rev.* 2014; 5: CD009405. http://doi.org/10.1002/14651858.

Hughner RS, Kleine SS. Views of health in the lay sector: A compilation and review of how individuals think about health. *Health.* 2004; 8(4): 395–422.

Illich I. *Limits to Medicine, Medical Nemesis: The Exploration of Health.* Harmondsworth: Penguin; 1976.

Kelner M, Wellman B. Health care and consumer choice: Medical and alternative therapies. *Soc Sci Med.* 1997; 45(2): 203–12.

Kilby CJ, Sherman KA. Lay beliefs. In: Gellman M, editor. *Encyclopedia of Behavioral Medicine.* New York: Springer; 2018. https://doi.org/10.1007/978-1-4614-6439-6_101997-1.

Lai DW, Surood S. Chinese health beliefs of older Chinese in Canada. *J Aging Health.* 2009; 2(1): 38–62.

May C, Allison G, Chapple A, Chew-Graham C, Dixon C, Gask L, Graham R, Rogers A, Roland M. Framing the doctor-patient relationship in chronic illness: A comparative study of general practitioners' accounts. *Sociol Health Illn.* 2004; 26(2): 135–58.

Morgan M. The doctor-patient relationship. In: Scambler G, editor. *Sociology as Applied to Medicine*, pp. 55–70. London: Elsevier Health Sciences; 2008.

Morgan M. Hospitals and patient care. In: Scambler G, editor. *Sociology as Applied to Medicine*, pp. 71–82. Edinburgh: Saunders Elsevier; 2008.

Nettleton S. *The Sociology of Health and Illness.* 2nd ed. Cambridge: Polity Press; 2006.

Parsons T. *The Social System.* London: Tavistock; 1952.

Reminick RA. The evil eye belief among the Amhara of Ethiopia. *Ethnology.* 1974; 13(3): 279–91.

Renzaho AMN, Romios P, Crock C, Sønderlund AL. The effectiveness of cultural competence programs in ethnic minority patient-centered health care – A systematic review of the literature. *Int J Qual Health Care.* 2013; 25(3): 261–9.

Rothstein WG, Rajapaksa S. Health beliefs of college students born in the United States, China, and India. *J Am Coll Health.* 2003; 51(5): 189–94.

Roussou E. Believing in the supernatural through the 'evil eye': Perception and science in the modern Greek cosmos. *J Contemp Rel.* 2014; 29(3): 425–38.

Scambler G. Health and illness behaviour. In: Scambler G, editor. *Sociology as Applied to Medicine*, pp. 41–54. London: Elsevier Health Sciences; 2008.

Silverman J, Kurtz S, Draper J. *Skills for Communicating with Patients.* Boca Raton: CRC Press; 2016.

Singer M, Baer H *Introducing Medical Anthropology: A Discipline in Action.* New York: Altamira Press; 2007.

Szasz TS, Hollender MH. A contribution to the philosophy of medicine: The basic models of the doctor-patient relationship. *Arch Intern Med.* 1956; 97(5): 585.

Taber JM, Leyva B, Persoskie A. Why do people avoid medical care? A qualitative study using national data. *J Gen Intern Med.* 2015; 30(3): 290–7.

Waskul DD, Eaton M. *The Supernatural in Society, Culture and History.* Philadelphia: Temple University Press; 2018.

Wilding JP, Mooney V, Pile R. Should obesity be recognised as a disease? *BMJ.* 2019; 366: doi: 10.1136/bmj.l4258.

Zhao M, Esposito N, Wang K. Cultural beliefs and attitudes toward health and health care among Asian-born women in the United States. *J Obstet Gynecol Neonatal Nurs.* 2010; 39(4): 370–85.

Zola IK. Medicine as an institution of social control. *Sociol Rev.* 1972; 20(4): 487–504.

CHAPTER 2

The body as a social entity

....

ABSTRACT

Mrs Annie Griffins and her husband visit a fertility centre to enquire as to whether they can schedule the conception of their baby and select its sex. Also, Mrs Griffins wants to know how she can gain her slim figure back after giving birth. Mrs Griffins's case is an example of various sociological terms, such as regulating bodies, individual, social, and politic body, cyborgs, authoritative knowledge, embodiment, the body as a project, and medicalisation. This chapter aims to help healthcare students and practitioners appreciate how the body is not merely a physical but also a social entity, through which people build their social identity and their understanding of the social world, and work with patients in a sensitive manner.

LEARNING OBJECTIVES

- Describe the processes through which the body is not merely a physical entity but a societal product as well.
- Explain the following terms:
  - Individual, social, and politic body.
  - Cyborgs.
  - Regulation of bodies.

DOI: 10.1201/9781003256687-3

- Embodiment.
- The body as a project.
- Explain medicalisation and give examples.

Note: Think about or discuss the questions that are in boxes before you continue reading through the chapter.

SCENARIO

Annie and George Griffins are in their early 30s, and live in the United States. They married a year ago and are looking forward to having a baby. Ideally, they want to have two children: two boys. They believe that they should have absolute authority over their bodies and be able to decide on the issue. They searched the internet extensively and found out they can indeed determine the sex of their children and are excited by this prospect. As a result, they visit a famous fertility centre located in their home-town in New Jersey, to explore the issue further. The relevant doctors inform Annie and George that there is no such technology at the centre which could help them choose the sex of their child. The doctor did not recommend it anyway and suggested trying naturally.

DISCUSS

1. Why do Mr and Mrs Griffins want to choose the sex of their child?
2. Which sociological concepts are relevant?
3. What further information do you need from the literature in order to answer these questions?

THE INDIVIDUAL, SOCIAL, AND POLITIC BODY

What Annie and George want to do brings to light various sociological concepts that need further scrutiny. Annie and George were born and raised in the United States; it is a Western industrial society, which is technologically advanced and places particular emphasis on individual control and success (Giddens, 2006; Messner and Rosenfeld, 2013). They wish to have complete control over nature and to choose the sex of their children, thereby turning Annie's body into a machine that can be programmed according to human desire and demand. Scheper-Hughes and Lock's (1987, p. 6) approach can be used to explain Annie's attitudes and behaviour towards her body. More specifically, Annie's body may be viewed in three ways: *first*, it can be 'individual', which means that she has a strong awareness of her body and wishes to have full control over it. Featherstone and Hepworth (1991) stressed that contemporary societies placed emphasis on lifestyle and planned ways of life, whereas Kelly and Field (1996) argued that the body served as the vehicle for forming an individual's identity. Therefore, self-control and control of the body are important elements in the process of projecting the body to the social world for acceptance and recognition. *Second,* Annie's body is 'social' because it receives specific social meanings, which are created in the context of choosing the sex of her child. Her body becomes a machine that is programmed to produce specific outcomes. In other words, Annie's body works like a metaphor, which actually symbolises a contemporary society where machines (cars, computers, telephones, factory machines, etc.) prevail and are under the control of human beings. *Third*, Annie's body is 'politic' because it is under social control and is regulated (e.g., by the media, education, and medicine) to be an autonomous body and to use advanced technology to achieve its goals. On this basis, the body is considered normal and acceptable in modern society.

In addition to the social aspects of Annie's body, the baby that Annie and George want to have acquires a new socio-technological status. That is, it becomes a 'cyborg baby'. Davis-Floyd and Dumit (1998, p. 1) described cyborgs as 'symbiotic fusions of organic life and technological systems', asserting that cyborgs derive from the use of technology to control one's life and to surpass natural forces. Along similar lines, Mitchell and Georges (1998) argued that the fetus became a cyborg by ascribing to it meanings which were infused by the use of technology. Interestingly, though a cyborg baby may be Annie's creation, the use of medical technology may end up backfiring as it ascribes identity to fetuses and presents them as independent agents (Rothman, 1994). For example, using technology (during ultrasounds) doctors often portray fetuses as playing, dancing, waving their hands, and so forth. Within this framework, fetuses acquire rights, which are often against the parents' will, plans, and power (Heriot, 1996; Franklin, 2001). Even though Annie thinks that she has the right to control her body and her baby with the help of technology, technology can create a cyborg baby that can stand alone and convey the message that Annie should not really have the power to design a male or a female.

Annie and George exhibit such attitudes towards selecting the sex of their child because they have been socialised with values that stress the importance of self-control, body ownership, individual success, and autonomy, which have shaped their social identity and have had an impact on their way of thinking. In Bourdieu's (1991, p. 12) terms, these values have become their second nature and inform their 'habitus', which causes them to interpret their world accordingly. It is these embodied values that have determined Annie's 'modes of attention' (Csordas, 1993) in such a way so as to feel that she can control fertility and the sex of her child. It would be interesting to see whether these modes of attention could be diverted towards what Annie and George can actually control (e.g., having intercourse without the use of contraceptives), thus allowing them to accept the fact that they cannot currently choose the sex of their child.

FURTHER DEVELOPMENTS

After the visit to the clinic, Annie and George continued searching for any possible information that would make their dream of having two boys a reality, but they could not find anything reliable. So, they decide to conceive naturally. Annie becomes pregnant three months later and both she and her husband are delighted; however, they also have a sense of uncertainty about the matter. They visit a gynaecologist, Dr James Addison.

Dr James: Hello! I am Dr Addison. You must be Annie and George. What brings you here? I hope you have good news!

Annie: We think so. My period is late, about one month now. I took a pregnancy test a couple of days ago and it was positive.

Dr James: That's very good! Why don't you lie down on the examination table and let's see what an ultrasound will show us.

Annie: Excuse me, Doctor, but are you going to examine my vagina?

Dr James: No, not this time.

Annie does not like the abrupt answer but, for the time being, she just wants to know if she is indeed pregnant and if everything is fine.

Dr James: Today, we will see your baby.

Annie: So soon? How is that possible?

Dr James: Well, I use the ultrasound machine over your belly and the fetus will show up on the screen.

Annie: So, you will be able to see inside me?

Dr James: Not exactly, I will use the machine to get a visual of the inside of your abdomen and uterus.

> *Dr James Addison starts describing scientifically what he observes inside Annie's body. At this stage, Annie finds the whole description, and even her body, as being very alien to herself since she cannot comprehend what Dr Addison is explaining; all she sees is the inside of her body as it appears on a black and white screen, which she cannot interpret. Suddenly, she hears the baby's heartbeat and is excited.*

Annie: Is this my baby?

Dr James: Yes, and everything looks and sounds just fine.

Annie: Doctor, we do not want to know the sex of our child. We want to find out when the baby is born.

Dr James: No problem, you won't find out from me! You just need to be careful and avoid lifting weight; you need lots of rest. I also want you to take some vitamins and folic acid supplements, which I am prescribing to you now.

> *Annie and George do not want to know the sex of their child. They want to hold onto the hope that, once the baby is born, it will be a boy. They think that if they find out now that they are having a girl that they will feel disappointed throughout the pregnancy and, possibly, develop negative feelings towards the baby. However, if, when their child is born, they find them-selves with a little baby girl then they may instantly accept that.*

DISCUSS

1. What social issues arise from this consultation?
2. What further information do you need from the literature in order to answer this question?
3. How could the doctor better approach the patient?

THE REGULATION OF BODIES

Annie finds Dr James Addison's attempt to examine the fetus inside her body highly intrusive, while his scientific explanations and her body suddenly become foreign to her. By stating, 'I will look inside your abdomen and uterus', Dr Addison shows that he understands and treats the body as a purely biological entity and he describes what he sees through terms used in natural sciences (Toombs, 1993). For Dr Addison, Annie's body is a separate entity, while Annie regards herself and her body as one and the same. Interestingly, after hearing her body discussed in medical terms, Annie starts viewing it as alien too and separate from herself.

Annie's experience is a manifestation of the 'regulation of bodies' in modern society. The regulation of bodies refers to the process of attempting to control bodies and human behaviour by certain individuals in power through various methods such as knowledge and technology (Turner, 1992, p. 210; Hall, 2001; Cregan, 2006; Ettorre and Kingdon, 2012). More specifically, Turner (1992) argued that the regulation of bodies was observed in various social institutions such as the law, religion, education, and medicine. Goffman (1957) called these organisations 'total institutions', which exerted a holistic control over the inmates. Within these institutions, the inmates were devoid of social roles, they did not own anything, they were forced to adopt behaviours and bodily postures, they did not have any private space and they were under surveillance and could not freely have social relations. The regulation of bodies goes back to Foucault's (1977, p. 170) analysis of modern medicine and society. Foucault used the term 'disciplinary power' to describe the situation in which bodies were controlled, changed, and corrected, such as in prisons and hospitals. Within such contexts, new knowledge was generated by scrutinising the bodies.

Annie finds herself in her gynaecologist's office, which operates according to very specific rules as to how the body should be monitored. That is, the pregnant body is controlled by the doctor and medical technology, while the pregnant woman does not have the freedom to choose how her body should be monitored, within the context of medical knowledge and technology (Davis-Floyd and Sargent, 1997). Within obstetrics, more specifically, Annie's body goes through three different sites of disciplinary power. *First*, Annie's body is observed by Dr Addison using medical technology. This is what Foucault (1977, pp. 170–94) called 'hierarchical observation'. *Second*, Annie's body goes through a 'normalizing judgement' by being measured and assessed according to standards. In this case, the size of the fetus, the rate of its heartbeat, and the position of the placenta are all examined and assessed. *Third*, Annie's body is scrutinised and fixed within what Foucault called 'examination'. This is done through the offering of medical advice and required medication that will support a gestation period that is free of any complications.

According to Foucault (1980), the regulation of bodies started in the 18th century when the size of the population in Western societies increased dramatically and the need to control large populations arose. As a result, bodies were regulated and became subject to intervention, should they have deviated from predetermined standards. Turner (1992) maintained that the state substituted the Church in its role of monitoring people's bodies and life. Within this sociohistorical context, the concept of the general hospital developed, and doctors dominated the system of healthcare. Zola (1972), more specifically, explained that medicine was an institution of social control, which was achieved by both the hegemonic position of doctors and by the process of medicalisation of biological phenomena that previously were not under the scrutiny of medicine. Zola stipulated that the medicalisation of society may occur at four levels. *First*, many aspects of life that are beyond biological functioning, such as lifestyle and habits, are increasingly placed under medical observation and are subject to improvement. *Second*, medical professionals increasingly acquire more and more legitimate control over people's bodies due to advancement in medical technology and research. *Third*, due to this increasing control, doctors now have access to areas that used to be understood as private. For example, doctors can examine and heal the inside of a person's body. *Fourth*, medicine is increasingly taking corrective actions towards people's health, lifestyle, and habits. Conrad (2007) adds two more factors which have given rise to medicalisation. *First*, social movements very often exert pressure on the medicalisation of conditions or behaviours. For example, Alcoholics Anonymous (AA) contributed to the medicalisation of alcoholism. Here, Conrad pointed out the role of laypeople (i.e., people without medical training and background) and their eagerness to have a condition medicalised and, thus, treated scientifically. *Second*, the competition between specialisations and professions escalated the medicalisation process, as an attempt to prove who possessed the most appropriate scientific knowledge. In this case, Conrad used the example of pregnancy and childbirth and the rise in competition between obstetricians and midwives.

Medicalisation is a process which, according to Conrad and Schneider (1980), consists of five stages. Initially, a behaviour may be considered as socially deviant even before a medical approach is given to it. In the next stage, there is an attempt to study the behaviour scientifically and, subsequently, a relevant study appears in a scientific journal. At this stage, a medical view of the behaviour is developed. From that point onwards more studies may shed further light on the deviant behaviour so as to present it as an urgent subject for intervention. Then, the request for intervention may be legitimised by the authorities. In the final stage, the behaviour or the condition is listed under the medical taxonomy, and intervention programmes or therapies are designed and implemented. This process is not linear, and it may start at different stages or include fewer stages. To illustrate, Conrad (2007) provided the example of how male baldness was medicalised through the initial involvement of medicine as the agent which scientifically labelled baldness as a male problem. Consequently, the involvement of media culture and the portrayal of baldness as an unattractive male image prompted men's negative stance towards it. The interplay of these agents led to a unified approach to baldness, which resulted in its full medicalisation – that is, scientific understanding and treatment.

Another interesting example, which illustrates Conrad and Schneider's stage of medicalisation, is that of the medicalisation of obesity. Although during the Renaissance a fat body was associated with wealth and beauty (Dawes, 2014), nowadays it is measured, classified, and linked with ill health, and shame. The Body mass index (BMI), which measures weight in relation to height (i.e., division of weight in kilograms by height in metres squared), classifies people to underweight (18.5 or less), normal weight (18.6–24.9), overweight (25–29.9), and obese (30 or above) (Lopez-Jimenez and Miranda, 2010). What has contributed to this shift is the meanings the relevant labels carry and the process of normalising standard weight (Brown, 2015). More specifically, 'overweight' implies that there is a 'right' weight to be achieved; hence people have to have it as a life target. 'Obese' is even more problematic because it comes from the Latin word 'obesus', which means 'having eaten until fat' (Brown, 2015). Such meaning points out individual action, responsibility, and accountability. Apart of the labels, the institutionalisation of obesity started in the late 19th century when physician Luther Emmett Holt published length and weight standards in his 1894 book *The Care and Feeding of Children*. Such standards were the predecessor of the BMI (Dawes, 2014). Later, in the 1940s, according to Brown (2015), a life insurance company set up a table of the standard weight in North America, which essentially caused Americans to start reconceptualising their bodies and comparing them with reference points; eventually comparing them with other people. In 1949, the National Obesity Society was founded aiming to focus on the treatment of obesity. Although obesity was treated as a problem in the 20th century, it was not until 2013 that it was officially declared a disease by the American Medical Association (AMA). Interestingly, the AMA assigned the review of the issue to its own Committee on Science and Public Health, which suggested that obesity should not be considered a disease because it did not fit the definition of a disease and there were people whose BMI was in the obese category, yet they were very healthy. Despite this, the AMA officially recognised obesity as a disease. The reasons for the decision largely related to management procedures and insurance reimbursement in the sense that a declared disease would capture more research attention, doctors would be reimbursed for treating it, and people would be eligible for specialised treatment (Brown, 2015). The issue is still debated today. On the one hand, based on medical and epidemiological data, obesity has been associated with serious conditions, such as type II diabetes, cardiovascular, as well as mental illness (Ciciurkaite, Moloney, and Brown, 2019; Syed, 2019; Rosen, 2014). On the other hand, counter arguments highlight that obesity is only a risk factor; some obese people are very healthy and declaring obesity as disease is likely to take autonomy away from and disempower people (Wilding, Mooney, and Pile, 2019).

Returning to our case, Dr Addison has medicalised Annie's pregnancy and the fetus. He has framed the female body and the fetus in a manner in which they are seen as imperfect machines, which need monitoring by medical technology and support through medication. Ragone and Willis (2000, p. 308) suggest that the medicalisation of childbirth was observed in three ways. *First*, 'conceptually' Annie's pregnancy is defined as abnormal, vulnerable, and in need of medication (through the vitamins and folic acid). *Second*, 'institutionally' Annie's vulnerability is legitimised since it is diagnosed by legally accepted medical professionals. *Third*, the medicalisation of Annie's pregnancy occurs through the relationship she has already formed with Dr Addison, in which he is the expert with whom Annie consults. In line with this third mode of medicalisation, Jordan (1997) outlined the example of a pregnant woman in a labour room whose knowledge of pregnancy and the fetus did not count. Jordan used the term 'authoritative knowledge' to explain that knowledge in a labour room was hierarchical, starting at the top with the physician's knowledge. Cartwright (1998) studied electronic fetal monitoring (EFM), a process which measured the baby's heartbeat and uterine contractions and was used in order to take necessary corrective actions. EFM served as an example of how modern technology could assist in producing knowledge and normalising pregnancy and gestation.

As Annie's experience in the labour room shows (below), physicians usually do not have direct contact with pregnant women and the woman's body is separated into the 'interactive end' and the 'business end' (Jordan, 1997, p. 69). The interactive end, which is the upper end of the body, interacts with the nurse in terms of what she is expected to do, whereas the 'business end', consisting of the abdomen and the vagina, is under the control of the physician. In such a relationship, medical technology is often used to reinforce and validate a physician's position and, thus, solicit hierarchical knowledge. Although Dr Addison could not un-medicalise Annie's pregnancy, based on basic clinical communication skills (Silverman, Kurtz, and Draper, 2016) he could have approached her in a sensitive manner by explaining the process of examining her, obtaining consent at the beginning and throughout the process, and showing understanding of Annie's concerns or her views about her body.

FURTHER DEVELOPMENTS

In the fifth month of her pregnancy Annie sees some blood and she instantly thinks that she has lost the baby. She immediately visits her doctor, Dr Addison, and is relieved when he assures her that everything is fine with her baby. However, not everything is fine with the pregnancy. In fact, the placenta is located too low in the uterus and Annie has to be very careful and rest a lot so that she does not go into miscarriage. Annie takes Dr Addison's advice very seriously; she makes sure to rest and she manages to keep the baby and herself safe until she gives birth.

She goes into labour in the 42nd week of gestation. As soon as she arrives at the clinic, the nurses ask her to lie on the examination table and wait for her doctor to arrive. Annie finds that all the procedures are conducted in a manner that is fast, intrusive, and inhumane. She does not say anything, however. At this point, she is in pain and is attending to her body.

Annie: Why does it hurt so much? I want the baby out now; I can't take the pain anymore!

Dr James: Don't worry, Annie. Your baby will be here soon. I will need you to push when I tell you to, OK?

Annie: Don't tell me what to do! Just get this baby out of me.

Dr James: Alright, Annie. It's time to push. Now, push!

Annie is now in severe pain, and she has stopped listening to the doctor.

Dr James: Annie, if you do not cooperate with me now then the baby will not be able to come out.

Annie: Really, Doctor? How on Earth did women have babies in the past before obstetricians like you were around?

Dr James: Just push now, Annie ...

> *The baby suddenly becomes stuck, and Dr Addison is worried about this development. Then, the rate of the baby's heartbeat drops, causing Dr Addison to order the nurses to prepare for an immediate Caesarean section.*

> *Annie gives birth to a healthy baby girl. George, Annie's husband, is happy with the outcome but is still somewhat disappointed that his child is not a boy. He tells himself that this is just an initial feeling that will go away in time. Annie wakes up a short while later and, when she learns about the sex of the baby, does not react. However, she bursts into tears later that day. She simply cannot accept her baby, her experience, her body, or the pain she is experiencing post operation. George does his best to calm her down.*

Annie: I am so sad.

George: Why?

Annie: Because the baby is a girl. It's just not what we wanted, right?

George: Yes, but it is our baby, and we will love her no matter what sex it is.

> *Annie is silent.*

George: Annie, we can't play God here.

Annie: Do you understand that this girl is responsible for me gaining 30 kilos? I cannot even imagine breastfeeding her. These breasts are mine, not hers!

George: No, sweetheart. It is not the baby's fault that, due to some complications during your pregnancy, you needed to stay in bed for a long period of time.

Annie: I don't care! It does not change the fact that I had to have a Caesarean, I gained 30 kilos and I now have a baby girl.

George: Why don't you think of it differently? You just gave birth to a healthy baby girl; you are healthy and more beautiful than ever.

Annie [bursts out]: I don't want this body; it is fat and ugly. I want my thin body back.

George: But Annie, you were not that thin before getting pregnant.

Annie: Yes, but I was almost there. I had been trying so hard to lose weight through my diet and my exercise regime.

DISCUSS

1. What new social issues are raised in the labour room and the conversation above?
2. What does Annie mean when she says that she wants her body back?
3. Why is this information important for doctors?

RITE OF PASSAGE, EMBODIMENT, AND THE BODY AS A PROJECT

Giving birth is like a rite of passage. Van Gennep (1960) explained that a rite of passage was a transition from one stage to another, before an individual acquired a new social status (e.g., adulthood, marriage). Such a process consisted of three main stages, made up of 'separation' from the social world followed by a 'transition' and, later on, 'incorporation' into the social world. Annie is removed from the social world when she is accepted into the clinic to give birth. In the labour room, Annie is in transition, between being a pregnant woman and becoming a mother. In this transitional stage, as Van Gennep argued, the person is confused and carries no identity. Similarly, the status of Annie's body and self are ambiguous, without fixed physical and social functions. Annie's body is separated into two parts: the upper end, which is attended to by the nurse and the lower end, which is seen to by the doctor. Annie's self is put on hold for the duration of the delivery and what matters is Annie's body, which is turned into a machine that executes two different tasks that each requires specific attention. The doctor focuses on the lower part of her body, which largely relies on the upper part for the smooth delivery of the baby. Thus, the self becomes an object for medical advice and guidance and, if it fails to cooperate, is then considered as a bad object, or as a diseased object that may require further medical intervention in order to transform it into a good object (i.e., helping the woman to relax or performing a Caesarean). In other words, during delivery, Annie's body is medically constructed as good or bad. Annie's self and body should acquire a more stable social status when the delivery is over, and she is free to return home and to her habitual daily activities. But, in Annie's case, her transition seems to continue for a long time after the delivery because Annie has difficulty accepting her new body.

A systematic review and meta-synthesis by Hodgkinson, Smith, and Wittkowski (2014) showed that women were concerned and dissatisfied with their body image after giving birth and thought that their identity was compromised because their understanding of themselves as mothers did not accord with their role as wives or partners. Hodgkinson, Smith, and Wittkowski carried on explaining that women's view of their bodies did not reflect what the society expected, and they wished they could regain their thin bodies. Annie believes that she is fat and ugly, and she feels like her breasts have become independent entities, which exist solely for her baby and not for her.

Interestingly, an earlier study by Upton and Han (2003) found that women who had given birth found themselves alienated from their breasts because they felt as though they had lost control over their breasts. That is, their breasts were now there to serve a different purpose, namely, to satisfy their baby and not themselves. In order to regain control over their bodies, women took certain decisions regarding what to wear and what to eat. However, a woman's perception of her body does not change easily because societies ascribe meanings to the body, causing her to act on the basis of these meanings. In other words, if a certain body shape is socially undesired, the person's identity is negatively affected. Annie finds that the 30 kilos she gained has contributed to her body image, and this makes her feel bad about herself. As she is in the initial stages of the post-partum period, she simply cries and shouts because she wants her body back. Put differently, using Douglas's (1966, p. 35) terms, Annie's new body is a 'matter out of place'. Annie does not accept her new body because it no longer meets socially acceptable standards. Annie's body is no longer in line with social rules and, thus, Annie attributes this deviation to her pregnancy.

Annie's behaviour indicates that she has embodied the social values of modern society, which were communicated by various social institutions, such as her peer groups, family, the media, and so on, as well as her experience of pregnancy and giving birth. She then interprets her embodied experience of pregnancy and birth in accordance with the embodied cultural and social values of what is considered as the acceptable female body. Merleau-Ponty (1962) argued that people's experiences are embodied and that we cannot function without such embodiment. Thus, our body is 'lived' (Toombs, 1993, p. 51). We, as bodies, have intentions to act and we are aware of what we can do rather than what we are (Toombs, 1993). Annie, based on Toombs's theoretical tenets, experiences pregnancy and birth as an illness, in the sense that she cannot be social and do the tasks that she used to do. For example, she cannot wear the clothes she used to wear when her body was thin. Annie's body, interestingly, becomes an undesirable object that is alienated from her. Moreover, Annie used to take her body for granted and regarded it as an integral part of her. Thus, she never attended to it until she felt the baby inside her and felt the pain during delivery and after her surgery. It is under such experiences that the body becomes present and acquires its status as an independent entity.

Annie's behaviour towards and her beliefs about her body image are reminiscent of Shilling's (1993, p. 5) term, the 'body as a project', which means that a person's body has not yet been completed and that a person continues to work on their body until they achieve a desirable version of it. Annie explains to her husband that her pre-pregnancy body was not as thin as she would have liked it to be, but she was working on making it thinner. In other words, achieving a thin body was, according to Annie, a life project that was close to completion. As a result of her pregnancy, Annie's aim of having a thin body was now a faraway goal and she would have to start all over again in order to achieve her goal. Based on Shilling's approach, understanding the body as a project provides Annie with the feeling of having control, which she lost due to her pregnancy and her post-partum body.

FURTHER DEVELOPMENTS

Annie is devastated. Two days have passed. She has not yet seen her baby and refuses to do so. Dr Addison visits her and tries to change her mind without success. George decides to take a more drastic approach and brings the baby downstairs to Annie's room without her permission. He has accepted the fact that he now has a girl, and he has decided that Annie has to do the same should they want their family to be united. However, things have become complicated with Annie as many undesired issues have suddenly merged – having a girl instead of a boy, gaining weight, having a Caesarean operation, and feeling pain after the procedure. However, George's strategy works well. Annie was caught by surprise when she saw her daughter, but when she held her in her arms, she was moved.

REFERENCES

Bourdieu P. *Language and Symbolic Power.* Cambridge, MA: Harvard University Press; 1991.

Brown H. *Body of Truth: How Science, History, and Culture Drive Our Obsession with Weight – And What We Can Do About It.* Philadelphia: Da Capo Lifelong Books; 2015.

Cartwright E. The logic of heartbeats: Electronic fetal monitoring and biomedically constructed birth. In: Davis-Floyd R, Dumit J, editors. *Cyborg Babies: From Techno-Sex to Techno-Tots*, pp. 240–254. New York: Routledge; 1998.

Ciciurkaite G, Moloney ME, Brown RL. The incomplete medicalization of obesity: Physician office visits, diagnoses, and treatments, 1996–2014. *Public Health Rep.* 2019; 134(2): 141–9.

Conrad P. *The Medicalization of Society: On the Transformation of Human Conditions into Treatable Disorders.* Baltimore, MD: John Hopkins University Press; 2007.

Conrad P, Schneider JW. *Deviance and Medicalization: From Badness to Sickness.* St Louis, MO: Mosby; 1980.

Cregan K. *The Sociology of the Body.* London: Sage; 2006.

Csordas TJ. Somatic modes of attention. *Cult Anthropol.* 1993; 8(2): 135–56.

Davis-Floyd RE, Sargent CF. Introduction: The anthropology of birth. In: Davis-Floyd ER, Sargent CF, editors. *Childbirth and Authoritative Knowledge: Cross-Cultural Perspectives*, pp. 1–51. Berkeley, CA: University of California Press; 1997.

Dawes L. *Childhood Obesity in America: Biography of an Epidemic.* Cambridge: Harvard University Press; 2014.

Davis-Floyd R, Dumit J. Introduction: Cyborg babies – Children of the third millennium. In: Davis-Floyd R, Dumit J, editors. *Cyborg Babies: from Techno-Sex to Techno-Tots*, pp. 1–20. New York: Routledge; 1998.

Douglas M. *Purity and Danger: An Analysis of Concepts of Pollution and Taboo.* New York: Praeger Publisher; 1966.

Ettorre E, Kingdon C. Reproductive regimes: Governing gendered bodies. In: Kuhlmann E, Annandale E, editors. *The Palgrave Handbook of Gender and Healthcare*, pp. 162–177. 2nd ed. London: Palgrave Macmillan; 2012.

Featherstone M, Hepworth M, Turner BS. *The Body: Social Process and Cultural Theory.* London: Sage; 1991.

Foucault M. *Discipline and Punish: The Birth of the Prison.* New York: Pantheon; 1977.

Foucault M. *Power/Knowledge: Selected Interviews and Other Writings 1972–1977.* New York: The Harvester Press; 1980.

Franklin S. Biologization revisited: Kinship theory in the context of the new biologies. In: Franklin S, McKinnon S, editors. *Relative Values: Reconfiguring Kinship Studies*, pp. 302–320. Durham: Duke University Press; 2001.

Giddens A. *Sociology.* 5th ed. Cambridge: Polity Press; 2006.

Goffman E. Characteristics of total institutions. In: *Symposium on Preventive and Social Psychiatry.* Washington, DC: Walter Reed Army Institute of Research; 1957.

Hall S. Foucault: Power, knowledge and discourse. In: Wetherell M, Taylor S, Yates SY, editors. *Discourse Theory and Practice: A Reader*, pp. 72–81. London: Sage; 2001.

Heriot MJ. Fetal rights versus the female body: Contested domains. *Med Anthropol Q.* 1996; 10(2): 176–94.

Hodgkinson EL, Smith DM, Wittkowski A. Women's experiences of their pregnancy and postpartum body image: A systematic review and meta-synthesis. *BMC Preg Childbirth.* 2014; 14(1): 1–11.

Jordan B. Authoritative knowledge and its construction. In: Davis-Floyd RE, Sargent CF, editors. *Childbirth and Authoritative Knowledge*, pp. 55–79. Berkeley, CA: University of California Press; 1997.

Kelly MP, Field D. Medical sociology, chronic illness and the body. *Sociol Health Illn.* 1996; 18(2): 241–257.

Lopez-Jimenez F, Miranda WR. Diagnosing obesity: Beyond BMI. *AMA J Ethics.* 2010; 12(4): 292–8.

Merleau-Ponty M. *Phenomenology of Perception.* New York: Routledge; 1962.

Messner SF, Rosenfeld R. *Crime and the American Dream.* 5th ed. Belmont: Wadsworth; 2013.

Mitchell LM, Georges E. Baby's first picture: The cyborg fetus of ultrasound imaging. In: Davies-Floyd R, Dumit J, editors. *Cyborg Babies: From Techno-Sex to Techno-Tots*, pp. 105–124. New York: Routledge; 1998.

Ragone H, Willis SK. Reproduction and assisted reproduction technologies. In: Albrecht GL, Fitzpatrick R, Scrimshaw SC, editors. *The Handbook of Social Studies in Health & Medicine*, pp. 308–320. London: Sage; 2000.

Rosen H. Is obesity a disease or a behavior abnormality? Did the AMA get it right? *Mo Med.* 2014; 111(2): 104.

Rothman BK. *The Tentative Pregnancy: Amniocentesis and the Sexual Politics of Motherhood.* 2nd ed. London: Rivers Oram Press/Pandora; 1994.

Scheper-Hughes N, Lock MM. The mindful body: A prolegomenon to future work in medical anthropology. *Med Anthropol Q.* 1987; 1(1): 6–41.

Shilling C. *The Body and Social Theory.* London: Sage; 1993.

Silverman J, Kurtz S, Draper J. *Skills for Communicating with Patients.* Boca Raton: CRC Press; 2016.

Syed IU. In biomedicine, thin is still in: Obesity surveillance among racialized, (im) migrant, and female bodies. *Societies.* 2019; 9(3): 59.

Toombs SK. *The Meaning of Illness: A Phenomenological Account of the Different Perspectives of Physician and Patient.* Dordrecht: Kluwer Academic Publishers; 1993.

Turner BS. *Regulating Bodies: Essays in Medical Sociology.* London: Routledge; 1992.

Upton RL, Han SS. Maternity and its discontents: 'Getting the body back' after pregnancy. *J Contemp Ethnogr.* 2003; 32(6): 670–92.

Van Gennep A. *The Rites of Passage.* London: Routledge & Kegan Paul; 1960.

Wilding JP, Mooney V, Pile R. Should obesity be recognised as a disease? *BMJ.* 2019, 366. doi: 10.1136/bmj.l4258.

Zola IK. Medicine as an institution of social control. *Sociol Rev.* 1972; 20(4): 487–504.

CHAPTER 3

The experience of chronic illness and disability

ABSTRACT

Mr George Maros is a Greek migrant who resides in Manchester and suffers from end-stage kidney disease. He is 40 years old and married with three children who are 5, 8, and 15 years old. He has a managerial position at a bank and works long hours, while his wife teaches at a Greek school in the Greater Manchester area. Due to his chronic condition, he has to visit the haemodialysis department at a local hospital three times per week in order to filter and clean his blood. During his visits he typically discusses his experiences with the nurses and shares his story with the other patients. George's tale illustrates a number of sociological terms such as the sick role, biographical disruption, the negotiation model, and illness narratives. The chapter aims to help healthcare students and practitioners to appreciate the impact of a chronic condition on their patients' lives, and to work with them in a sensitive and supportive manner.

LEARNING OBJECTIVES

- Explain why chronic illness is a social experience.
- Describe the social changes a chronic patient goes through.
- Explain the following terms: sick role, biographical disruption, negotiation, coping strategy and style, illness narratives and normalisation, disability.

DOI: 10.1201/9781003256687-4

> Note: Think about or discuss the questions that are in the boxes before you continue reading through the chapter.

SCENARIO

Mr George Maros has been recently diagnosed with end-stage kidney disease and, therefore, he has to undergo dialysis treatment until an organ is available for transplantation. Initially, he was shocked and scared by his prognosis. After taking some time to process the situation, he now feels sad but, more importantly, stressed as he feels uncertain about his future. He shares his sentiments with Ms Judith Maclean, a nurse at the haemodialysis department.

Judith: Good morning, what is your name? You must be a new visitor.

George [in a low, dull voice]: Yes. My name is George.

Judith: You don't seem very well, George. Is there anything we could do for you?

George: Can you give me my health back?

> *Judith is taken aback by his question.*

Judith: We can do our best to provide you with the best treatment possible.

George [angrily]: That's not enough! [*George pauses for a moment and collects himself.*] I am sorry; it is not your fault. I am just very disappointed, frustrated, stressed, and worried.

Judith: I understand. You have just been diagnosed with a chronic illness and, naturally, you will need some time to understand what the disease is and what haemodialysis is.

George: The only positive thing seems to be that no one blames me for what has happened to me. This makes it easier for me to avoid some of my daily activities and devote this time to seeking medical treatment. I just hope that an organ is found soon so that I can undergo the transplantation and, once I am healthier, return to my normal routine and lifestyle.

Judith: I think you simply need to give yourself some time to get used to it.

George: I feel that I have a dysfunctional body which prevents me from living my life the way I am used to. For example, I can't work as many hours as I used to since I have to be here three times a week for about five hours each time. Also, I won't be able to travel abroad or out of town for work, which I am required to do in order to maintain my salary. And on a more personal level, I can't play with my children, take holidays ... Basically, I feel as though my life as I know it is over.

Judith: It is a big change. I assure you that we will be here to support you in every possible way.

George: Unfortunately, I can't work. Who is going to manage my department while I am away? I really worry about this affecting my job and, in turn, my ability to be a good husband, father, and provider for my family. I am really worried about how all this will impact my life.

Judith: In my experience with other patients, everything works out alright. It might be difficult at the beginning, but you will see that you will find ways to deal with any kind of disruption you might face.

George: We'll see how it goes.

Judith smiles and leaves the dialysis room.

DISCUSS

1. What new role is George expected to perform?
2. Why does George have feelings of anxiety and sadness?
3. What social changes is George facing?
4. What further information do you need from the literature in order to answer these questions?

THE SICK ROLE AND BIOGRAPHICAL DISRUPTION

George has a new social role now. This is what Parsons (1952) identified as 'the sick role', which refers to a series of rights and obligations a person has once biomedicine diagnoses the presence of a chronic illness. According to Parsons, illness is a form of deviance because the patient is no longer able to perform daily activities as efficiently as before. However, the patient is not deemed responsible for what has happened and is excused for withdrawing from social activities. Interestingly, this is a temporary state, in the sense that the patient should wish to become well and, thus, is expected to seek out medical help in order to restore health and return to social activities.

George has end-stage kidney disease, which is socially considered to be a form of deviance in the sense that the disease makes George deviate from his normal social role as a worker, parent, and consumer. However, George is not reprimanded for the disease and is not considered responsible for having end-stage kidney disease in the first place. Thereafter, he might be treated in a special way by society. On the other hand, George has some obligations. He is expected to withdraw from work and social activities, look for medical help to improve his condition and, following this, return to his previous work and social activities. In other words, it is legitimate for George to take on a temporary role so as to restore his normal social life.

The notion of the sick role has been criticised by many scholars. Varul (2010) argues that the concept of the sick role is not currently used as a framework for explaining chronic illness as the experience of chronic illness is very complex and is influenced by many institutionalised acts, such as the marketisation of health, medicalisation, patient reinforcement and support, and so forth. The complexity of illness experience was identified in early criticism which arose from Freidson (1970), who explained that entering the sick role was not universal and should not be taken for granted. He outlined three types of legitimate access to the role. *First*, there are cases in which the patient gets well quickly because the disease is curable and, thus, does not have to go through all the stages associated with the role. *Second*, in cases in which a patient suffers a lethal disease, the cycle of the sick role cannot be completed because the patient cannot really take any action in order to overcome their illness. *Third*, in cases in which the disease is a stigmatising condition (e.g., AIDS), societies may not expect, or encourage, the person to assume the sick role and seek help in order to return to a normal social life.

Freidson's criticism is valid and the legitimacies he describes show that the sick role is much more complex than was outlined by Parsons. However, George's case seems to further support at least some aspects of the sick role as conceived by Parsons. More specifically, end-stage kidney disease is not curable, but it has a healthier turning point, which is kidney transplantation. This means that George is temporarily regarded as sick until an available organ will enable him to stop undergoing haemodialysis and will allow him to return to his regular social activities. So, society validates for George to assume the sick role for as long as it takes to obtain a new kidney. Moreover, end-stage kidney disease is not a deadly disease, though life expectancy is much lower than that of healthy people (Ojo et al., 2001; Oniscu et al., 2005). Given that kidney transplantation is a possibility, George is justified in entering the sick role and taking action. Finally, legitimate access is strong in George's case because end-stage kidney disease has not been associated with personal conduct and, thus, no responsibility lies on the patient's shoulders for having brought on the disease. In other words, end-stage kidney disease is not a stigmatising condition and society excuses George for withdrawing from work and social activities and expects him to reach out for medical assistance.

Within the sick role, George experiences various social changes. He explains to the nurse that he cannot work the long hours he used to, and he may not be able to support his family or fulfil social obligations as before. The changes that George is going through are described by what Bury (1982, p. 169) named 'biographical disruption', which refers to the disruption to, or upheaval of, one's identity or what they understand as a normal social life. Using Bury's terminology, biographical disruption happens at three levels in George's case. *First*, George experiences the disruption of what he took for granted. The long working hours, travelling for work, and holidays, which were routine activities for George, are now at risk. *Second*, George's biography is disrupted. George has constructed a very successful biography over the years by participating in social institutions. He has been a successful manager, a husband, a father, a consumer, and so forth. Now, all these contexts that he has come to identify himself with are under threat. As such, George worries because his sense of self-integrity and control are threatened, and George associates this with the fear of the changes that are imminent. *Third*, George tries to respond to disruption by reconsidering and activating former social networks. He is lucky to have so many friends he can rely on, and he anticipates that their support will alleviate his disruption. He is also planning to reactivate his network of chess players and resume a tournament among his friends. He thinks that this will keep him active, and it will provide him with a cause in which he can participate and maintain the respect of his peers. Despite the fact that George acknowledges the limitations of activating social resources – such as not being able to fulfil the obligations involved with such social participation – he aims to put his social network into use.

However, George is not only concerned with his biographical disruption but also with the meanings that his disease possibly encompasses (Bury, 1997). That is, end-stage kidney disease has consequences for George's life, which actually means that the disease is perceived as a separate entity on the one hand. On the other hand, it gradually becomes part of George's self because the self is restricted and, thus, acquires a new identity over time – that of the 'disabling self'. Bury (1997) pointed out another meaning that is associated with the disabling self, which refers to the symbolism associated with the disease. In the case of George, the disease may be associated with the terms 'unproductive' and 'inactive', especially for a person who is 40 years old and is used to being socially active and successful. In other words, the symbolisation of social restriction does not accord with the social expectations of a 40-year-old man. Such symbolisation has led George to view himself as half-human, as he explains below.

FURTHER DEVELOPMENTS

Judith enters the dialysis room after about two hours and finds George feeling a sense of uncertainty once again.

Judith: How are you feeling now, George?

George: To tell you the truth I feel strange, almost alien. It is hard to believe that my blood is being removed from my body and is being passed through these tubes in order to be 'washed' in this huge machine.

Judith: Oh, George! You have such an imagination. Of course, you are still human. It's good of you to use humour to try to come to terms with the situation.

George: I'm not trying to be funny. I'm being rather serious; connected to the machine in this way makes me feel almost inhuman. I've become half-human!

Judith: What do you mean George?

George: I am simply half of my former self. I need a machine to survive and so I cannot be as social or physically active as before.

DISCUSS

1. What social aspects does the term half-human entail?
2. What could be done in order for George to overcome the feelings he is currently experiencing?
3. What further information do you need from the literature in order to answer questions 1 and 2?

FURTHER DEVELOPMENTS

George has been undergoing dialysis treatment for six months now. He seems to have become used to the process but still feels sad and uses the term half-human to describe himself. One day, he explains his feelings to another patient, Andrew, who occupies the bed next to George. Judith passes by and happens to overhear George's testimonial.

Judith [looking at Andrew]: George likes to use humour. Of course, he is a human being. He just likes making fun of himself.

George: Pay no attention to her; this is exactly how I feel. I have told her many times that I can't stand having my life separated into two parts: my body and the machine. I feel that, on account of this disruptive and time-consuming treatment, I cannot live a full life and so I am half-human.

Andrew: I understand what you mean. I actually feel the same way.

Judith is embarrassed. She feels as though she tried too hard to be empathic and support George to overcome his negative view of his body and his self, but George's attitude has not changed. Instead, he has begun influencing other patients to develop similar attitudes.

George: It is more than that. I have to undergo dialysis during Christmas and other holidays when people are with their friends and relatives. While others are enjoying their time, I have to be here surrounded by people, without any privacy. We are all dressed the same, as though we are prisoners. I am 40 years old, but the majority of patients are older. It seems that I am among the youngest and I feel that I should not be here. Nobody would expect someone my age to suffer from this disease. I am sure that the other patients take pity on me and are thinking to themselves how lucky they are to have been diagnosed at an older age.

BODILY AND SOCIAL INTEGRITY, AND DISABILITY

The term half-human has been used by dialysis patients on the island of Cyprus (Constantinou, 2012). Constantinou interviewed patients who experienced both dialysis and kidney transplantation. He found that dialysis patients, especially those who were between 20 and 60 years old, described haemodialysis as a torturous process and themselves as half-human. This description reflected on two aspects of their selves. *First,* the self was split into two parts: the self and the machine. So, an alien or technological part became integrated with the former self in order for the patient to survive. Thereafter, the need for technology affected the person's integrity. *Second*, the restrictive character of dialysis (a process that is completed three times per week for four hours at a time) led the patients to feel as though they had become half of their former social selves, whereby they could not fulfil their normal social obligations and, thus, might not be as respected as before.

Dialysis patients, similar to George, did not only regard themselves as half-human since they could not fulfil all their social obligations but also because their social life was generally disrupted. For example, George had to have dialysis during the Christmas holidays, when other people spent time with their friends and relatives. Due to the time commitments imposed by the dialysis process, George's sociality is constantly disrupted, and this leads to growing frustration. Moreover, George finds himself in a stigmatising context, where the majority of patients are older than him. He believes he stands out from the crowd and, consequently, feels bad about being ill at such a young age. The issues of stigma and stigmatisation are thoroughly explored in Chapter 4.

Interestingly, Constantinou (2012, p. 36) found that patients who had had kidney transplantation emphasised how free they felt as they no longer had to undergo dialysis and, as such, described themselves as becoming 'proper' human beings once again. The word 'proper' (σωστός), as used in Cyprus, denotes two meanings, which were embedded in the patients' words. *First*, proper means whole and reflected on the fact that patients did not need a machine in order to survive, so they restored their self and bodily integrity. *Second*, proper means being right or being able to fulfil social obligations. In the Cypriot context, where social obligations are considered very important, a person who is able to fulfil their social obligations (i.e., towards their family and peers) thereby receives the respect of their community.

Constantinou's findings on end-stage kidney disease and bodily integrity capture the social aspects of disability. There are two main models of defining disability and its underpinning ramifications, namely the medical model and the social model (Barry and Yuill, 2016). Based on the medical model, disability is a form of bodily impairment which results in restrictions in the person's life. This means a medical condition is present and is causing challenges to the ill person. Focusing on the medical condition, responsibility for change lies with the healthcare system to provide therapies and management regimes, and the individual to adhere to therapy, while the individual is left alone to meet other non-medical needs, such as work and leisure. Such an approach ignores the social context or any structural factors which cause an impairment to be even more restricting and limiting for the individual (Williams and Busby, 2002).

The social model shifts attention from the individual to society. That is, disability results from the restrictions placed by society on the person who has an impairment. Therefore, it is not necessarily a spinal injury, for example, that causes an individual who is in a wheelchair to be disabled but the poor infrastructure in a society that does not provide opportunities for easy access to services in the community. The social model has many more ramifications than the medical model in the sense that it reaches out to encompass the society as a whole, from infrastructure, to services, to social attitudes and biases, and so forth. As a result, the social model has informed policies and laws for equality, diversity, discrimination, disability benefits, etc. As Williams and Busby (2002, p. 175) put it,

> if disability is seen as a personal tragedy, disabled people are treated as individual victims of unfortunate circumstances. If disability is a form of social oppression, disabled people can be seen collectively and the victims of an uncaring, discriminating society, whose most effective remedy for their conditions is protest and resistance.

Although sometimes the medical and social models are in conflict, both of them are necessary for a more holistic understanding of the impairment in the individual's life. Kutner and Zhang (2017) found that there are people with end-stage kidney disease who are not able to work and that these people are more likely than their employed counterparts to suffer depression. Gołębiowski et al.'s (2020) study indicated that almost half of dialysis patients were disabled largely due to cardiovascular complications. They were not able to work, and they were dependent on other people. Reflecting George's feelings about the impact of the disease on his social life, Gołębiowski et al.'s study shows that kidney failure is not merely a problem of physical malfunctioning. It is also about how society responds to it and provides patients with opportunities to meet their daily and long-term needs, beyond healthcare.

FURTHER DEVELOPMENTS

A year has passed since George was diagnosed with end-stage kidney disease and he still refers to himself as half-human. However, he seems to have found a way to redefine his condition and lived experience. One day, while undergoing dialysis, he starts up a conversation with a new patient, Peter, who arrived at the haemo-dialysis department a week ago and seems confused and afraid.

George: I had the same feelings a year ago and was on the verge of depression. I used to describe myself as half-human because I was dependent on a machine, and I could not do the things I was used to doing. Well, I still feel that I am half-human sometimes because I still depend on a machine to survive. In general, though, I feel much better now.

Peter: What changed?

George: Well, mainly I believe it is the way that I think about things. I still work on a full-time basis and try to make up the hours I miss due to my dialysis over the weekends, especially when I have paper-work to do. Also, I focused more on my social life. I reactivated a chess tournament that I used to coordinate a few years ago. So, friends get together to compete and win a prize, which is a free one-week holiday to a European city. I also participate in patient groups and advise new patients who are in need of psychological support.

Peter: That's good to know. I think that I may need more time before I can take similar actions.

George: Yes, it always takes time. I have to say that my education and career have helped provide me with a template to use when it comes to my disease. As a manager at the bank, I have a habit of trying to inform and educate myself as much as possible about various issues and I used the same approach to this. I educated myself to the point where I felt that I could be the manager of my disease.

NEGOTIATION: COPING, STRATEGY, AND STYLE

Bury (1991, 1997) stressed that chronic patients find ways to respond to their condition and their new experience. They negotiate (Bury, 1997, p. 129) with their experience and new self, in order to accept the condition and find new meaning to their life. George still thinks that he is half-human due to his physical dependency on the dialysis machine, but he renegotiated with his new self and found ways to overcome his frustra-tion and uncertainty. He activated his cognitive mechanisms by com-paring himself with other dialysis patients and found that he is the one patient who works full-time. This has provided him with positive vali-dation and has encouraged him to keep working. Since he also advises other patients, his example of working full-time in spite of the illness serves as a prototype and as a good example for other patients. George's cognitive processes resemble what Bury (1991, p. 460) has termed 'coping'. Apart from the way in which George has interpreted his working status, George's behaviour reflects 'strategy' (Bury, 1991, p. 461), which refers to George's actions to deal with disruption. That is, he reactivated a chess tournament, and he participates in patient groups as an advisor to new patients. Such actions have helped George maintain a socially active lifestyle and, as a result, have led to an improvement in his sense of worth. George also uses specific approaches to respond to disruption and portray his illness experience and actions, in accordance with the term 'style' (Bury, 1991, p. 462). He basically draws from work and cultural values, such as education and management skills, in order to present his disease in a way in which he has become the manager of the disease. In other words, George uses the style of a manager to understand and handle living with end-stage kidney disease.

FURTHER DEVELOPMENTS

George describes his experience to many patients as he volunteers his time in order to share his story with members of patient groups. He explains how much he suffered from end-stage kidney disease and how things have improved over time. He places emphasis on the period during which he was diagnosed and how he was shocked initially and how he was overcome with fear and uncertainty and describes the physical and social restrictions he had to endure due to haemodialysis. He then tells them about the changes he made in order to cope with the disease and treatment and how he discovered new meanings because of his condition. He usually ends his talk by noting that he anticipates that once he has his kidney transplant he will no longer need dialysis and will be able to gain back his active body and self.

Another new patient, Sasha, wants to learn more about George's experience.

Sasha: George, tell me more about your haemodialysis experience. In all honesty, this is the aspect of the disease that I fear the most.
George: What can I say about having to undergo dialysis? Initially, when I was diagnosed, I was shocked; almost depressed. It was a very difficult period. I started going to the centre for treatment in the mornings, and I've also tried going in the afternoon. Now, I think I might

try the night shift. I find it harder to do the treatment during the holidays and over the summertime. But then I think to myself that there are other people who work on a shift basis, who work during the night, or very early in the morning, as well as over Christmas and other holidays. I think of other people who might be in a similar position as me and that gives me the strength to carry on.

Sasha: That's a good way to look at it. In any case, you are right; we are not in a more disadvantageous situation compared to other, healthier people.

George: Yes. I sometimes tell people that I have a permanent job as a bank manager, and that I also have a part-time job as a haemodialysis patient three times a week. Unfortunately, the part-time job does not pay much! [*Laughs*]

Sasha: It is remarkable that you can use humour when describing your experiences.

George: Actually, I tell my close friends that I'm visiting my girlfriend, also known as the dialysis machine, when I come here. [*Laughs*]

DISCUSS

1. What does George actually do when he describes his experience? Can you identify any patterns?
2. What are the functions of his storytelling?
3. Does George use different types of storytelling?

ILLNESS NARRATIVES AND NORMALISATION

George does not merely describe his experiences with end-stage kidney disease and haemodialysis. Instead, he actually tells a constructed story of what he went through and how he interpreted his encounters. George's descriptions are carefully selected and organised in such a way as to construct a coherent story, with a specific plot. That is, diagnosis leads to suffering (haemodialysis), which in turn is followed by adaptation and, finally, kidney transplantation. George's constructed, narrated story is an example of Kleinman's (1988, p. 49) definition of illness narrative, which refers to 'a story a patient tells, and significant others retell, to give coherence to the distinctive events and long-term course of suffering'. The plot helps the story acquire entity, which alludes to a destined experience George has, starting from the disease and suffering and ending with kidney transplantation and the restoration of social life. George's strategic way of building his story is reminiscent of Williams's (1984, p. 178) approach to a narrative. That is, a narrative has the 'routine' side, in which patients put an event in order, and the 'reconstructed' side, which refers to a process through which patients reshape their narratives in order to explain the cause of their disease.

The question here is why is George constructing such a story? The answer has been well researched and is addressed in the relevant literature. More specifically, Kierans (2005) argued that illness narratives helped patients maintain stability in their daily life and participate in social activities; Garro and Mattingly (2000) stressed that narration gave meaning to patients because the process of creating a narrative involved cognitive and social mechanisms, while, at the same time, cultural values and resources were mobilised (Arduser, 2014). Furthermore, illness narratives function as a therapeutic framework for patients because they help patients express themselves and allow them to be heard. Garro and Mattingly (2000) have outlined additional functions; a narrative builds a picture for the audience. Citing Austin, they stressed that a narrative did not only tell things, but it also did things. That is, narration is a form of doing, and patients may act according to their story in order to provide their audience with some evidence. Hunt (2000) maintained that narratives helped people redefine their condition and their experiences in order to accommodate their feelings of frustration and uncertainty. Moreover, Reissman (2000) explained how patients placed emphasis on the importance of specific aspects of their social life so as to compensate for the loss of others. Interestingly, Mattingly (2000) argued that narratives possessed a plot; that is a beginning, a middle, and end, with the aim of constructing a coherent tale. Coherence made the story easier to communicate with and be listened to.

George does not merely construct a consistent plot; instead, he uses different forms of narration. *First*, he compares himself with other healthier individuals and realises that having haemodialysis during the Christmas holidays should not be regarded as a disadvantage as healthy people may also have to work on these days. In other words, George's sociality is not more restricted than other people's. He is basically using a narrative of equality. *Second*, he compares having haemodialysis with having an extra, part-time job or like having a secret extramarital affair. By doing so, he relies on the narrative of normalisation through which he presents haemodialysis as routine and common. Normalising directly relates to equality because, by presenting one's condition as routine, one places oneself on an equal basis with other, healthy people who have routinised their lives.

Normalisation happens in a two-fold manner, which relates to telling and acting. George's way of normalising his condition is on a par with the modes of normalisation described by Amelang et al. (2011, p. 61), who studied normalisation practices in three European countries among patients who had had organ transplantation. They found that patients normalised their condition in two main ways. *First,* patients, like George, normalised their condition by redefining and narrating their experience. Here, 'ideologies' had an impact on the way in which patients reconsidered their body and their selves. *Second,* they changed their activities in such a way as to bring back their daily routines (e.g., they were engaged in sports). Amelang et al. explained that these actions were heavily influenced by medical guidelines or discourses. In this case, George took actions to reactivate a chess tournament and participated in patient groups as a patient counsellor following Judith's advice.

Normalisation as action has also been scrutinised by Charmaz (2000), who argued that normalising was a means to control one's disease symptoms, illness, and life. It could also alleviate the effects of stigma because other people no longer understood the condition as alien or strange since it was now a routine. Thus, routinisation could serve to make the condition one that a patient is more likely to accept. Charmaz (2000) explained that there were two types of normalisation that relate to patients' actions. *First,* the condition is normalised without the patient's awareness. This happens when patients act without an aim to normalise the condition (e.g., attributing a condition to normal biological changes). *Second,* the changed body and self become familiar and, thus, are routinised over time. For example, a dialysis patient who accepts that haemodialysis is part of their life, with the passing of time.

Keeping in mind all of his descriptions, George began with the 'chaos' narrative when he was uncertain, afraid, and frustrated and could not see any benefits from such an experience. At the time, while narrating to Judith, he sounded completely lost and threatened. George used other types of narratives, too. He used the 'restitution' narrative (Frank, 1995, p. 115) by describing his suffering, the diagnosis, and his attempts to deal with the disease. He also used the 'quest' narrative by arguing that he learned a great deal from his experience (he learned how to appreciate small things and how to help others, for example) (see also Llewellyn et al., 2014; Diver, Avis, and Gupta, 2013). In addition, George's narratives are also reminiscent of the victim, survivor, and heroic narratives (Kirmayer, 2000). He understood himself as a victim because he was too young to have end-stage kidney disease but, over time, he survived and did much better than other patients as he was able to keep working on a full-time basis. All the types of narratives that George utilised perform specific functions, mainly, to make his story and himself more appealing to others and, thus, more acceptable.

FURTHER DEVELOPMENTS

Upon reflection, Judith realised that trying to empathise and be supportive was not enough and could have led to a negative relationship between a health professional and their patient. To begin with, healthcare professionals need to understand the experience of chronic illness; what patients go through; show interest; give patients time and space; what they do in order to cope with their condition and their life changes; how they tell their story, and why it is so important for patients that their experience and their story are heard and valued. Following this, Judith raised the issue with the nursing manager and suggested that nurses and doctors should undergo training on how to interpret patients' actions and words, as having such skills would allow them to work more effectively and appropriately with diverse patients.

REFERENCES

Amelang K, Anastasiadou-Christophidou V, Constantinou CS, Johansson A, Lundin S, Beck S. Learning to eat strawberries in a disciplined way: Normalization practices following organ transplantation. *Ethnol Eur.* 2011; 41(2): 54–70.

Arduser L. Agency in illness narratives: A pluralistic analysis. *Narrative Inq.* 2014; 24(1): 1–27.

Barry AM, Yuill C. *Understanding the Sociology of Health: An Introduction.* 4th ed. London: Sage; 2016.

Bury M. Chronic illness as biographical disruption. *Sociol Health Illn.* 1982; 4(2): 167–82.

Bury M. The sociology of chronic illness: A review of research and prospects. *Sociol Health Illn.* 1991; 13(4): 451–68.

Bury M. *Health and Illness in a Changing Society.* New York: Routledge; 1997.

Charmaz K. Experiencing chronic illness. In: Albrecht GL, Fitzpatrick R, Scrimshaw SC, editors. *The Handbook of Social Studies in Health & Medicine*, pp. 177–292. London: Sage; 2000.

Constantinou CS. 'Now, I am a proper human being': Kidney transplantation in Cyprus. *Med Anthropol.* 2012; 31(1): 29–43.

Diver C, Avis M, Gupta A. Quest, chaos and restitution: The illness narratives of individuals diagnosed with fibromyalgia syndrome. In: Richards R, Creek R, editors. *Chronicity: Care and Complexity*, pp. 25–40. Brill; 2013.

Frank AW. *The Wounded Storyteller: Body, Illness, and Ethics.* Chicago, IL: University of Chicago Press; 1995.

Friedson E. *Profession of Medicine: A Study of the Sociology of Applied Knowledge.* Chicago, IL: University of Chicago Press; 1970.

Garro LC, Mattingly C. Narrative as construct and construction. In: Mattingly C, Garro LC, editors. *Narrative and the Cultural Construction of Illness and Healing*, pp. 1–49. Berkeley, CA: University of California Press; 2000.

Gołębiowski T, Kusztal M, Konieczny A, Letachowicz K, Gawryś A, Skolimowska B, Ostrowska B, Zmonarski S, Janczak D, Krajewska M. Disability of dialysis patients and the condition of blood vessels. *J Clin Med.* 2020; 9(6): 1806.

Hunt LM. Strategic suffering: Illness narratives as social empowerment among Mexican cancer patients. In: Mattingly C, Garro LC, editors. *Narrative and the Cultural Construction of Illness and Healing*, pp. 88–107. Berkeley, CA: University of California Press; 2000.

Kierans C. Narrating kidney disease: The significance of sensation and time in the emplotment of patient experience. *Cult Med Psychiatry.* 2005; 29(3): 341–59.

Kirmayer LJ. Broken narratives: Clinical encounters and the poetics of illness experience. In: Mattingly C, Garro LC, editors. *Narrative and the Cultural Construction of Illness and Healing*, pp. 153–180. Berkeley, CA: University of California Press; 2000.

Kleinman A. *Rethinking Psychiatry: from Cultural Category to Personal Experience.* New York: The Free Press; 1988.

Kutner NG, Zhang R. Ability to work among patients with ESKD: Relevance of quality care metrics. *Healthcare (Basel).* 2017; 5(3): 42.

Llewellyn H, Low J, Smith G, Hopkins K, Burns A, Jones L. Narratives of continuity among older people with late stage chronic kidney disease who decline dialysis. *Soc Sci Med.* 2014; 114: 49–56.

Mattingly C. Emergent narratives. In: Mattingly C, Garro LC, editors. *Narrative and the Cultural Construction of Illness and Healing*, pp. 181–211. Berkeley, CA: University of California Press; 2000.

Ojo AO, Hanson JA, Meier-Kriesche H, Okechukwu CN, Wolfe RA, Leichtman AB, Agodoa LY, Kaplan B, Port FK. Survival in recipients of marginal cadaveric donor kidneys compared with other recipients and wait-listed transplant candidates. *J Am Soc Nephrol.* 2001; 12(3): 589–97.

Oniscu GC, Brown H, Forsythe JL. Impact of cadaveric renal transplantation on survival in patients listed for transplantation. *J Am Soc Nephrol.* 2005; 16(6): 1859–65.

Parsons T. *The Social System.* London: Tavistock; 1952.

Riessman CK. 'Even if we don't have children [we] can live': Stigma and infertility in South India. In: Mattingly C, Garro LC, editors. *Narrative and the Cultural Construction of Illness and Healing*, pp. 128–152. Berkeley, CA: University of California Press; 2000.

Varul MZ, Parsons T. The sick role and chronic illness. *Body Soc.* 2010; 16(2): 72–94.

Williams G. The genesis of chronic illness: Narrative re-construction. *Sociol Health Illn.* 1984; 6(2): 175–200.

Williams G, Busby H. The politics of 'disabled' bodies. In: Calnan M, Gabe J, Williams SJ, editors. *Health, Medicine and Society*, pp. 185–218. London: Routledge; 2002.

CHAPTER 4

Labelling and stigma

··

ABSTRACT

Mrs Mary Christian receives complaints from friends and close relatives that she has been very distant lately and that she has isolated herself from everyone. They initially think that Mary is depressed, possibly due to personal unresolved issues or problems with her husband. When they confront her with this, Mary reacts angrily and intensely, eventually demanding that they leave her alone because she thinks that her friends and relatives do not care about her anymore. Mary seeks help from her GP because her diabetes is out of control due to feeling stressed all the time. Her GP refers her to a psychologist who, upon further consideration of Mary's experiences and descriptions, ends up concluding that Mary's stress results from experienced stigma. This chapter aims to help healthcare students and practitioners to maintain genuine interest in exploring their patient's story and to appreciate the impact of stigma on their patients' lives.

LEARNING OBJECTIVES

- Outline the main principles of the labelling and stigma theory.
- Define the terms blemishes of individual character, abominations of the body, and tribal stigma.
- Explain the situations discredited, discreditable, and visibility and obtrusiveness.

DOI: 10.1201/9781003256687-5

- Describe the terms enacted, felt, and courtesy stigma.
- Outline how people may respond to stigma.

Note: Think about or discuss the questions that appear in boxes before you continue reading through the chapter.

SCENARIO

Mary Christian receives complaints from friends and close relatives that she has been very distant lately and that she has isolated herself from everyone. They initially think that Mary is depressed, possibly due to personal unresolved issues or problems with her husband. When they confront her with this, Mary reacts angrily and intensely, eventually demanding that they leave her alone because she thinks that they do not care about her anymore.

DISCUSS

1. What could be the reasons that Mary has socially isolated herself?
2. Why do you think she has been offended by the intervention led by her friends and family?
3. What questions would you construct in order to be able to classify Mary's behaviour?

FURTHER DEVELOPMENTS

Mary's friend, Anna, managed to approach Mary when she was in a better mood and recommended that she should consider visiting a psychologist. While Anna expected her friend to reject this idea, instead, Mary calmly responded, 'I know; that was my plan anyway. I will see my GP first. I am stressed and I am not sure why; I cannot even manage my glucose levels; my diabetes is out of control, and I am concerned'. Her GP, Dr Sean Parkins, referred her to a psychologist because he thought it was important to get to the bottom of Mary's psychological symptoms in order to better support her in managing her diabetes. Mary then proceeded to arrange an appointment with Dr Chris Menes. During their first visit, Dr Menes tried to gauge Mary's behaviour:

Dr Chris: Why do you no longer want to have contact with your friends?

Mary: Because I do not want to go to places which are crowded.

Dr Chris: Is it because you find such places noisy, tiring or …?

Mary: I suppose it is because I don't like the same things that they like anymore.

Dr Chris: Can you provide me with an example of something or some activity that they like, which you no longer enjoy?

Mary: Well, they like visiting kids' play areas, going to the mall, attending events, those sorts of things.

Dr Chris: And you don't like these activities because you don't have any children?

Mary: I do have a child, a four-year-old son!

> *Dr Chris Menes initially thought that Mary might be suffering from agoraphobia, a psychological disorder characterised by feelings of anxiety when one is in public spaces, which they feel that they cannot escape from. However, he was not sure if this was the case since Mary seemed to insist on being unable to attend places that attracted a lot of children, even though she herself had a child.*

Dr Chris: Mary, since you have a child, wouldn't it be better if you visited such places with your son?

Mary: Doctor, this is exactly what I try to avoid.

Dr Chris: What do you mean? What exactly are you trying to avoid?

Mary: Going out with my child.

Dr Chris: Why?

Mary: My child has Down syndrome and I feel that when we go out together people look at us. They think that my child and I are freaks. At the park, other children do not want to play with my son; their parents do not even talk to me. This is extremely hurtful, and I do not want this to continue. I can't help it, but I sometimes feel ashamed about having a child with Down syndrome. Sometimes I think that my child feels ashamed, too.

> *Dr Chris Menes is now convinced that agoraphobia is not the underlining cause of Mary's behaviour. Instead, her behaviour could be attributed to stigma.*

DISCUSS

1. Why has Dr Menes ruled out agoraphobia?
2. What do you understand by the term stigma?
3. What further information do you need from the literature in order to answer these questions?

RULING OUT AGORAPHOBIA

Agoraphobia is ruled out as, in the case of Mary, her actions do not meet certain criteria in order for her to be diagnosed with the condition. According to Kelley (1973), in order to conclude that certain behaviour is not random, and that it carries identifiable reasoning, one needs to consider the following three questions:

1. Does Mary avoid visiting all public spaces?
2. Does Mary avoid visiting specific places?
3. Are there any other visitors who feel embarrassed or ashamed at the places that Mary frequents?

If the answer to (1) is 'yes' and to (3) is 'no' (e.g., she avoids all public spaces, but no other people experience similar feelings), it seems that there is something intrinsic that is wrong and perhaps Mary suffers from a psychosocial disorder such as agoraphobia. If the answer to (1) is 'no' (which means that Mary is embarrassed only when visiting specific places) and (3) is 'yes' (other people have similar experiences), it possibly means that the reasons are extrinsic. That is, there may be something wrong with the social environment, which causes Mary and other visitors to feel alienated. If the answer to (2) is 'yes' and (3) is 'no' (e.g., Mary avoids visiting specific places, but no other people avoid these spaces), we may consider that something in that specific context disturbs Mary.

DISCUSS

1. Based on the current case, how would Mary probably answer the questions above?
2. Do her possible answers help you understand why agoraphobia can be ruled out?

Based on the information provided, Mary would answer 'yes' to (1) and 'no' to (3), which would lead to the assumption that the reason is intrinsic (i.e., agoraphobia) and we would then need to look further into Mary's way of thinking and her psychological state. However, Mary provides us with extremely important information when she describes that she has no problem at all when she goes outside alone. Instead, the problem arises when her child, who has Down syndrome, is with her. To this end, the cause is not psychological but largely social. Thereafter, agoraphobia as an intrinsic factor is ruled out, and we should look deeper into other extrinsic factors that eventually have had a negative impact on Mary's psychological wellbeing. This extrinsic factor has to do with labelling and stigmatising social environments. That is, environments in which people reject or dissociate themselves from other people, on the basis of perceived health problems.

LABELLING AND STIGMA

Green (2009) explained that stigmas are not given; rather, they are constructed and identified through six steps. *First,* labelling occurs in cases where conditions or characteristics are noted and, thus, are ascribed labels that represent these conditions. *Second,* behind the act of labelling is people's tendency to stereotype and, as a result, labels often carry negative stereotypes. *Third,* societies construct 'the other' and those labelled fall into the category of the other. This is a way to demarcate the boundaries between ourselves and the other and to compare the two groups, thereby devaluing the other in order to assign more value to ourselves. *Fourth,* societies understand those labelled as inferior. *Fifth,* labelled people are more likely to experience discrimination. *Sixth,* stigmas are constructed as a tool to be used by those in power to control the powerless.

Two terms that derive from the six steps of constructing stigmas, as outlined by Green, are labelling and stigma. Let me discern labelling first. Having a certain condition may be considered as a form of social deviance in the sense that it is a condition that most people do not have, and those who have it might not be able to perform the social activities that most people do. In case a person has a condition but the condition has not been labelled as deviance, it is a form of 'primary deviance' (Lemert, 1967, p. 17). It is identified as deviance because it differs from the social norm but is uncaught or unnoticed and, therefore, it does not have any social implications. In the event that others know, the condition is then classified as 'secondary deviance' (Lemert, 1967, p. 17) because it can now be labelled. A family with a child living with Down syndrome, as in the case of Mary, may be labelled as 'idiots' or 'retards', associating the child's condition with the rest of the family members. In a nutshell, labelling refers to the process of assigning a name to a condition or someone who has a condition. This name or label works as a cognitive template, guiding people's action.

However, how is a label assigned and by whom? Labels could be assigned by physicians at the stage of diagnosis (Green, 2009, p. 19). A diagnosis is a medical label, which represents a set of symptoms and a health condition. It is also a social label that may encompass the patient as a social actor. This is not to imply that physicians label people in order to discriminate against them. Rather, the labels used by physicians for diagnostic purposes may be used by societies as contexts of understanding humans as social beings. Furthermore, people may assign a label even in the absence of a medical diagnosis. This happens because people have preconceived notions of what does and does not constitute normal behaviour and characteristics. Anything that deviates from this may be considered as something that is foreign or alien, which needs to be controlled. Assigning a label, therefore, is a way to contain the unusual or the different, in the sense that it helps people to identify it and, consequently, better control it. In other words, the label serves to guide people's attitudes and behaviour. For example, a mentally ill person may behave in an unusual way, such as whispering or talking to themselves. Such behaviour can cause feelings of uncertainty among people who are not familiar with the mentally ill person's condition. Assigning a label to such a person, as aggressive, retarded, weird, and so forth, serves as a framework that allows people to understand the other person's behaviour and assume the required action – such as keeping a distance or being cautious around the person.

When labelling occurs, the deviant person may be stigmatised by other people. The term stigma represents a mark that results from labelling. It carries negative connotations, and it may dissociate the possessor of the stigma from other people. When attached, the stigma may 'spoil' the person's identity (Goffman, 1963), which means that the person may feel that the stigma dominates their life to the extent that they change their lifestyle and habits accordingly. Goffman (1963, p. 14) identified three main types of stigma. *First*, the 'blemishes of individual character' mean that a person's character possesses qualities that may be socially considered as weak or problematic. Mental disorders, addiction, and alcoholism are a few examples of the stigma of character. *Second*, the 'abominations of the body' refers to any bodily signs that may be devalued by society (e.g., a lower-limb amputee). *Third*, the 'tribal stigma' is a type of stigma that derives from a person belonging to a certain social group (i.e., race and religion).

Goffman (1963, pp. 57, 64, 66) stressed that stigma may be encountered by the stigmatised in three main social situations. These are: (1) discredited: others know and discredit the possessor of the stigma; (2) discreditable: others do not know but the possessor may be discredited if others know (in this situation the possessor is afraid of any disclosure about their conditions); (3) visibility and obtrusiveness: the stigma stands out more when in specific social contexts and interferes more with certain social interactions. For example, a person in a wheelchair at a party compared to a person in a wheelchair at a restaurant. In this example, mobility issues stand out more (more visible) at a party and people may be more likely to dissociate (more obtrusive) the person in the wheelchair with other people in a context where people are expected to dance.

Stigma also represents actions that the stigmatised person may experience (Goffman, 1963, pp. 15, 18; Scambler and Hopkins, 1986, p. 33). For example, stigma may be 'enacted' (i.e., the person may be discriminated against on the basis of the stigma) or 'felt' (i.e., the person internalises negative meanings about themselves). The stigmatised person may experience the 'courtesy' stigma (Goffman, 1963, p. 30) as well, where they are stigmatised because they are associated with a person who carries a discrediting mark. For example, the relatives of a person who has AIDS may be stigmatised because they are closely associated with the patient.

DISCUSS

1. Is the theory of labelling and stigma useful in accounting for Mary's behaviour?
2. If yes, apply the theory to explain her behaviour. If not, discuss possible alternative theories.

APPLYING THE THEORY OF LABELLING AND STIGMA TO MARY'S CASE

Mary finds herself in a situation in which her deviance is secondary given that her child's condition has been diagnosed and people are aware of it. However, Mary is afraid of carrying on in this secondary deviance situation, which could result in further stigmatisation and social dissociation. Mary's son has been experiencing both the enacted and felt stigma. He has been subjected to the enacted stigma because other children avoid playing with him in the park. Moreover, Mary's son has suffered the felt stigma because he has internalised negative ideas about himself and, subsequently, feels ashamed about his condition. Due to her association with her son, Mary has been stigmatised as well since other people avoid forming social relationships with her, experiencing the courtesy stigma in that way. Mary, therefore, does not want her child or herself to be subjected to this type of stigmatisation and prefers being under a discreditable situation where people do not know about her son's condition. To manage this, she avoids public spaces so that her child does not stand out (visibility) in a group of children who do not have Down syndrome and, moreover, is not further discredited (obtrusiveness) by children and adults who do not understand Down syndrome.

Mary's situation is no different from experiences that have been documented by social scientists who studied children with intellectual disabilities. Here, I rely heavily on Gray's studies of autism. In his article, 'Perceptions of Stigma: The Parents of Autistic Children', Gray (1993) explained that autism was a difficult situation for parents to cope with for a number of reasons. *First*, a child with autism might behave antisocially, which means that the parent might be held fully responsible for the control of the child. *Second*, the diagnosis of autism may take a long time and, consequently, may result in a frustrating experience. *Third*, a diagnosis might not be a relief for parents because the services available for children with autism were, at that time, not very well developed. *Fourth*, the public did not seem to have much knowledge about autism and this lack of knowledge might have negatively affected social reactions towards families with autistic children. *Fifth*, very few children with autism were expected to live on their own without support from relatives. Dealing with all these issues and raising a child with autism was a frustrating experience for parents who also endured stigma by association or affiliation with the child (what Goffman (1963) termed as the 'courtesy stigma').

The courtesy stigma describes a situation in which people feel stigmatised not because they have a condition but because they are closely associated with another person that possesses a stigmatising condition. For example, a parent with a child with mental disabilities is stigmatised because of their child's condition. The parent may be socially excluded and feel responsible for their child's condition or behaviour. Gray (1993) argued that parents of children with autism lived under a discreditable condition rather than under a discredited condition. This is due to the fact that parents had options for managing the public's awareness of their child's condition. Like Mary, they avoided going out with their child, they avoided using services, and shunned people that used very narrow definitions of normality. Further, in cases where the condition was not severe and the child looked normal, and families went unnoticed or passed as normal.

Gray (1993) set out to use this general knowledge gained from the literature to study and understand the experience of families with children with autism. He interviewed 32 parents – 23 mothers and 9 fathers – and found that the majority of these parents said that they were stigmatised in many respects. That is, raising a child with autism appeared to be a dominant experience and determined the parents' identity. In other words, raising a child with autism destroyed all other identities that the parent possessed, such as friend, employee, and so forth. One of the most difficult aspects for parents with autistic children was their restricted social life due to their child's condition. Thereafter, they confined their social activities to a few friends and some close relatives. When parents found themselves outside the house with their children pursuing leisure activities, they were concerned about dealing with their child's disruptive behaviour. The child's antisocial behaviour was problematic for parents in two main ways. *First*, children with autism might not have any physical characteristics that make their condition stand out. So, their behaviour does not accord with their physical appearance, and might result in intensified social reactions. *Second*, the public has high expectations from parents with autistic children and might blame them when they cannot control their child.

Another interesting finding by Gray highlighted that the child's condition was perceived to have had a negative impact on siblings, as siblings often had to take care of their autistic brother or sister and, as a result, they were stigmatised by their peers. Moreover, grandparents were also affected in the sense that they had their own understanding of their grandchild's condition and how it ought to be dealt with. Very often, grandparents and parents were in conflict with regards to the handling of the autistic child. Interestingly, Gray found that mothers were more likely to feel stigmatised than fathers; this difference the author attributed to the observation that mothers were more involved in raising the child and utilising the relevant services and, as a result, felt more responsible and were more socially exposed.

In a later study, Gray (2002) interviewed 53 parents in order to understand courtesy stigma among parents of children with high-functioning autism. Gray aimed to explore how courtesy stigma could be enacted or felt. To distinguish enacted and felt stigma in participants' answers, Gray (2002, p. 739) started the interviews with a rather structured question such as 'Do people treat you or your children differently because of your child's disability?' Parents were asked to name or describe specific encounters or experiences of being discriminated against due to their child's condition. In cases where parents could not describe specific experiences but shared the thoughts of other people concerning their child or themselves, their answers were classified under felt stigma. Gray found that most parents experienced felt stigma, which meant that they thought that they were stigmatised by other people. This was more prominent when they found themselves in public spaces where they had to deal with the child's disruptive behaviour. This also had to do with the fact that the child was more visible and, thus, more likely to be seen and stigmatised.

Nevertheless, parents experienced enacted stigma in some cases (Gray, 2002, pp. 740–1). The enacted stigma could take on three forms. *First*, they experienced 'avoidance' by other people, for example, when friends avoided inviting them to a party. This had an impact on the whole family, and especially on the child's siblings, who were in this way deprived of social interactions. *Second*, 'hostile staring by others' was also a form of the enacted stigma. This happened when the child's behaviour was socially inappropriate. *Finally*, parents of children with autism had to deal with 'rude comments by others'. This also happened due to the child's antisocial behaviour and the high social expectations of parents to keep their child in check. Gray explained that there were two facts that contributed to enacted stigma. That is, highly functioning children with autism were likely to be socially active, participate in social groups, and attend schools with children with no disabilities. This resulted in experiencing bullying and social isolation by their peers. In addition, the discrepancy between normal physical appearance and antisocial behaviour generated negative reactions from their peers.

Green's (2003) quantitative findings revealed interesting trends among 81 mothers of children with disabilities. That is, those mothers who understood people with disabilities as having been devalued by others were more likely to experience the courtesy stigma; their children were less likely to interact with normal children and more likely to interact with children with disabilities. These findings showed that mothers responded to perceived stigma by decreasing the visibility of the child's condition (by socialising with other children with disabilities) and, thus, reshaping the social expectations for both them and their child. Green et al. (2005) further explored the experience of families with children with disabilities by investigating Link and Phelan's (2001) classification of stigma. According to Link and Phelan (cited in Green et al., 2005), stigma has five elements. These consist of labelling (a difference is spotted and acquires social significance), stereotyping (the difference acquires negative social meanings), separation (the labelled person is dissociated from the others), status loss, and discrimination (the possessor's status in society is devalued and they experience discrimination). On the basis of these elements, Green et al. (2005) interviewed eight adults with disabilities and seven mothers of children with disabilities. It is worth noting that Green et al. found that people with disabilities were labelled due to their differences, and might be in a transitional state, in the sense that others did not know what to expect from them. In other words, their role and expected behaviour were not clear and were not classified. Furthermore, people with disabilities experienced stereotyping because others ascribed negative meanings to their difference or condition. Separation was another experience that people with disabilities had and they described cases in which others devalued them and excluded them from social relations. As a result of labelling, stereotyping, and separation, the participants of the study by Green et al. also experienced discrimination and loss of their status and sense of self-integrity when people dissociated from them.

Recent research has not produced any different results. More specifically, Watanabe et al. (2021) interviewed 23 parents with children with Down syndrome and found that parents experienced many types of courtesy stigma. That is, they experienced devaluing remarks and attitudes, social discrimination, stereotyping remarks, staring, social distancing, intrusive questioning, pitying remarks, and so forth. Parents tried to respond to courtesy stigma and employed an array of methods, such as concealing, social withdrawal, ignoring, being indifferent, information gathering, assigning meaning, asking advice, exploring options, educating others. Interestingly, Deakin (2014) found that children with Down syndrome may be more aware of their disability than previously thought and that they may also be aware of social reactions and stigma. Han et al.'s (2022) systematic review revealed that individuals with autism may experience various forms of stigma such as stereotypes, judgement, and discrimination and that they are well aware of this stigmatisation. Although autistic individuals may internalise stigma, they also respond in the following ways: concealing, selective disclosure, self-advocacy, reapproaching the situation, and understanding their identity in a positive way.

FURTHER DEVELOPMENTS

Dr Chris: Mary, have you done or tried anything specific to deal with the situation?

Mary: What could I do? This whole situation has made me very stressed. Sometimes I feel ashamed that I have a child suffering from Down syndrome.

Dr Chris: Alright. In these instances when you feel stressed, what do you do to make yourself feel better?

Mary: I don't know whether this is important or not but, in general, I try to dress my son in fashionable clothes so that he looks older and more mature. For example, I might have him wear a suit.

Dr Chris: Why do you do this?

Mary: Well, I am not sure how to say this ... but, I think that it makes him look different from the other children.

Dr Chris: Well, since that helps, then you should continue doing this. Is there anything else that you do that helps you in any way?

Mary: My son seems to enjoy swimming. I know that he is still very young, but I think he swims very well. Better than the other children who are healthy.

Dr Chris: OK, that's good for your son too!

Mary: You know, all this is a learning experience for me and my husband. I have learned how to become more patient and stronger in character. I know that I still need to work on how to deal with people and their attitudes and this is the main reason why I am here.

Dr Chris: Mary, do you feel that you can do things for yourself?

Mary: Well, yes and no. I still work, and I enjoy my work, but I do not have the same commitment that I used to have in order to evolve as an employee and pursue a proper career. I am too distracted and tired to do so.

DISCUSS

1. What does Mary do in order to deal with having a child with Down syndrome?
2. Why are Mary's strategies helpful for her?

RESPONSES TO STIGMA

Goffman (1963) explained that stigmatised people were not passive recipients of labels and stigmas. Instead, they responded to them and adopted various ways to deal with them. They might alter their body in a way that is more acceptable; they might place emphasis on other parts of the self, which were socially considered more valuable; they might present their experience as unique and stimulating and use their experience to explain their personal course. In essence, Mary uses all of these strategies. *First*, she dresses her child in a way that is different by making him wear a suit. In this way, other people may comment positively and focus on the pleasant appearance of the child, thereby avoiding or downplaying any physical or behavioural characteristics that pertain to Down syndrome. *Second*, she places particular emphasis on other aspects of her son's body, namely his physical ability to swim. She actually compares her son with other healthy children and notes that her son is a better swimmer compared to his healthier peers. In this way, Mary feels a sense of pride towards her son. *Third*, she presents her experience as stimulating and inspiring, in the sense that it has changed her way of thinking and her personality. In spite of the difficult situation, Mary feels strong enough to carry on, or at least stronger than other people who do not have to deal with such a situation. Once again, she compares her experience with that of other people and feels a sense of pride in raising a child with Down syndrome. *Fourth*, Mary excuses herself for not pursuing her career, as she would have done had she not had a child with Down syndrome. Such a strategy functions as a protective measure when faced with peer reviews and staff appraisals and, as a result, Mary feels more relaxed.

Interestingly, Link and Phelan (cited in Green, 2009) explained that people had difficulties responding to or dealing with stigma when they found themselves in relationships in which others had more power over the person who carried the stigmatised trait. However, it seems that modernisation has given people the ability to deal with stigma, which has been undergoing a shift towards a less effective framework. In her book, *The End of Stigma? Changes in the Social Experience of Long-Term Illness*, Green (2009) concluded that the stigma was still there, and people used it to devalue and control those that carried a stigmatised trait. However, it had gone through severe changes and its impact had been diluted due to changes at the technological, political, and personal level. That is, modern technology could potentially help a person with a chronic condition manage symptoms and any disruptions in their life. As a result, the person might be more likely than ever before to be understood as normal. At the sociopolitical level, a framework has been constructed in favour of people with differences or chronic conditions, in an attempt to realise the values of equality and human rights. Drawing from both the technological and political levels, people with chronic conditions might reconstruct their stories and narratives in a way that they feel they have control over their condition and are more likely to be accepted by others. Green concludes her book by stating that stigma is still powerful but, in recent times, it has come under attack. This attack may result in its further weakening in the future.

DISCUSS

1. Having identified the cause behind Mary's behaviour, what could Dr Chris Menes advise her to do in order to deal with stigma and the problem of avoiding public spaces?
2. What would you advise Mary to do?

FURTHER DEVELOPMENTS

In order to minimise the impact of stigma, Dr Chris Menes chooses to give Mary some simple advice, which will help her manage her concerns and, eventually, accept her child's condition. Thus, Dr Menes recommends that Mary try to go out more often and mingle with families that have children with Down syndrome.

Dr Chris: Mary, it is good that you have found your own way to deal with the situation, but I have a few other options to suggest.

Mary: What do you have in mind, Doctor? You cannot really change people. People have their own ideas and stereotypes about Down syndrome. You can't possibly change the attitudes and behaviours of individuals overnight?

Dr Chris: Certainly not. You could, however, influence people's attitudes and behaviour by changing your attitude and behaviour. If other people perceive that you are reserved and self-isolated because of your child's condition then you simply confirm their preconceptions and, thus, reinforce their actions. If you seem stigmatised, you basically solidify the boundaries of stigmatising environments. You need to break through such boundaries and dismantle stereotypes and biases.

Mary: That sounds good in theory, but how do I do this in practice?

Dr Chris: First and foremost, you need to accept the fact that you have a child with Down syndrome and keep in mind that this was through no fault of your own.

Mary: Well, I realise this, and I know that it will take me some time, but I will get there.

Dr Chris: Excellent! Given this acceptance, you need to get over the fear of being identified. Let others know about you and your child. Start going out more often and, in this way, you are basically facing your fear of disclosure.

Mary: Yes, but it is harder than it sounds.

Dr Chris: I know, but you need to make a start. It is easier to start going out if you socialise with other families with children with Down syndrome. If you do that then you create a context which is not stigmatising because your child is no different than the rest and so does not stand out in any way. When you socialise with these families over a long period of time, having a child with Down syndrome will be a very familiar situation for you; it will become second nature and you will start socialising in other contexts. By the time you socialise in other contexts, you will have the necessary skills to deal with other stigmatising situations. In the end, stigma will not have any use in your case because stigmas exist only if they have consequences. They have consequences when they manage to change the attitudes and behaviours of the person who is stigmatised.

DISCUSS

1. Why has Dr Chris Menes given this particular advice to Mary? What does he aim to achieve?
2. What main principles of the stigma theories does he rely on to formulate his advice?

EXPLAINING INTERVENTION

Dr Chris Menes wants Mary to open up, to start visiting social settings again, manage social reactions and, eventually, accept her child's condition and enjoy social interactions for the benefit of both her and her child. To achieve all this, Dr Menes encourages Mary to manage discreditability by presenting her child publicly and to decrease obtrusiveness by increasing her interactions with other families who have children with

Down syndrome. By doing so, Mary will deal with managing enacted, felt, and courtesy stigmas and, in turn, view herself on an equal footing with other people.

FURTHER DEVELOPMENTS

Dr Sean Parkins, Mary's GP, receives a full report about the causes of Mary's stress and he is pleased to read that Mary is now handling the situation better. Dr Parkins advises Mary to continue her current medication for diabetes before he gauges the situation again. Dr Parkins explains to his students, who have attended the consultation with Mary, that experienced stigma is a very problematic experience for patients because they may feel devalued, isolated, eat unhealthily, experience chronic stress which may cause hormonal changes, be physically inactive, not adhere to therapy, be distracted, and so forth. He stressed the importance for a doctor to have the necessary knowledge from social sciences and the communication skills in order to understand the situation early so that unnecessary medical examinations or conclusions are avoided. He carries on explaining that in the event he did not see that the issue was psychosocial he could possibly change Mary's medication unnecessarily, causing Mary to experience further uncertainty about the course of her diabetes.

REFERENCES

Deakin KA. *Perceptions of Down Syndrome: A Growing Awareness? Investigating the Views of Children and Young People with Down Syndrome, Their Non-disabled Peers and Mothers.* Doctoral dissertation. University of Glasgow; 2014.

Goffman E. *Stigma: Notes on the Management of Spoiled Identity.* London: Penguin Books; 1963.

Gray DE. 'Everybody just freezes. Everybody is just embarrassed': Felt and enacted stigma among parents of children with high functioning autism. *Sociol Health Illn.* 2002; 24(6): 734–49.

Gray DE. Perceptions of stigma: The parents of autistic children. *Sociol Health Illn.* 1993; 15(1): 102–20.

Green G. *The End of Stigma? Changes in the Social Experience of Long-Term Illness.* London: Routledge; 2009.

Green S, Davis C, Karshmer E, Marsh P, Straight B. Living stigma: The impact of labeling, stereotyping, separation, status loss, and discrimination in the lives of individuals with disabilities and their families. *Sociol Inq.* 2005; 75(2): 197–215.

Green SE. 'What do you mean "what's wrong with her?"': Stigma and the lives of families of children with disabilities. *Soc Sci Med.* 2003; 57(8): 1361–74.

Han E, Scior K, Avramides K, Crane L. A systematic review on autistic people's experiences of stigma and coping strategies. *Autism Res.* 2022; 15(1): 12–26.

Kelley HH. The processes of causal attribution. *Am Psychol.* 1973; 28(2): 107–28.

Lemert E. *Human Deviance, Social Problems and Social Control.* London: Prentice-Hall; 1967.

Link BG, Phelan JC. Conceptualizing stigma. *Annu Rev Sociol.* 2001; 27(1): 363–85.

Scambler G, Hopkins A. Being epileptic: Coming to terms with stigma. *Sociol Health Illn.* 1986; 8(1): 26–43.

Watanabe M, Kibe C, Sugawara M, Miyake H. Courtesy stigma of parents of children with Down syndrome: Adaptation process and transcendent stage. *J Genet Couns.* 2021; 31(3): 746–757.

CHAPTER 5

Mental illness

....

ABSTRACT

Mrs Chun Bowie is a migrant from China who moved to the UK 30 years ago. Though she never embraced modern medicine, she eventually decided to visit a local GP clinic as she had been suffering from tiredness and dizziness. She is initially interviewed by a medical student who concludes, after considering all the information he gathers from his patient, that Chun suffers from depression. His GP supervisor agrees with the diagnosis and informs Chun accordingly. Immediately, Chun refuses to accept the diagnosis and is now certain that modern medicine is not reliable or accurate. This chapter aims to help healthcare students and practitioners to appreciate the importance of the cultural understanding of mental illness and to work with patients in a shared decision-making process, under the umbrella of cultural competence.

LEARNING OBJECTIVES

- Explain the relationship between social class, gender, age, migration, and mental illness.
- Describe the main elements of the drift hypothesis and the opportunity and stress hypothesis.
- Explain the cultural influences on the way people understand mental illness.

DOI: 10.1201/9781003256687-6

> Note: Think about or discuss the questions that are in the boxes before you continue reading through the chapter.

SCENARIO

Mrs Chun Bowie is a Chinese migrant, living in the UK. She visits her local GP clinic because of symptoms of dizziness and fatigue. Chun had never truly embraced Western medicine and, initially, had tried alternative medicine to cure her symptoms. When this did not work, she decided to listen to a friend's advice and seek the help of Western medicine. She arranges an appointment with her local GP and now finds herself waiting to see the doctor. While waiting, she is approached by a senior medical student, Jason Krypton.

Jason: Hello, my name is Jason Krypton, I am a medical student and the GP asked me to talk to you before she sees you. Is that OK with you?

Chun is staring at the floor, and she slowly turns her head upwards to look at Jason. Her doubtful expression is discrediting for Jason, who is instantly disappointed but, nevertheless, continues talking.

Jason: I can see how this might be a tiring day for you. Is it OK if I take a short medical history from you? I will then inform the GP and she will contact you later for any pending issues.

Chun nods in agreement.

Jason: Before we begin, I wanted to assure you that anything you say will be treated confidentially. Is that OK?
Chun: Yes.
Jason: Thank you! What brings you here today?
Chun: I am tired and dizzy. I feel pain all over my body and I want some medication that will help me feel better. I have not slept for days.
Jason: Have you tried taking some painkillers?
Chun: Yes, but that did not help.
Jason: I see how this might be frustrating for you. Do you have any other symptoms?
Chun: No.
Jason: If you do not mind me saying, you seem somewhat sad. Is there anything in your life that makes you feel sad or upset?
Chun: No. I am just tired all the time.

Jason: What do you do in your free time? Do you have any hobbies?
Chun [smiles]: Well, I usually spend time at home, on my own.

DISCUSS

1. Has Chun visited the GP for any psychological issues?
2. What is Jason trying to identify through his questions?

FURTHER DEVELOPMENTS

Jason continues to collect information on Chun's past medical history, as well as information about her family history and her social lifestyle.

Jason: Mrs Bowie, how old are you?
Chun: I am 68 years old.
Jason: What do you do for a living?
Chun: I am a pensioner. I used to work in several places in the past, doing various jobs. I worked in a factory, and I also used to clean offices.
Jason: Do you currently face any financial difficulties?
Chun: How does that matter? I get a few pounds per month, enough to pay my rent, repay a loan, and sustain myself. I have enough to get by each month.
Jason: Do you have any friends or relatives nearby?
Chun: Well, I have my cat.
Jason: Do you have any children?
Chun: Yes, I have two grown sons who left the country a long time ago.
Jason: Where do you come from, Mrs Bowie?
Chun: I come from China. I moved to the UK 30 years ago and married a British man who died five years ago in a car accident.
Jason: It must be very difficult living on your own, away from your children and without your husband. It sounds like it could be a terribly lonely experience.
Chun: No, it isn't. As I said, I have my cat. Will you talk to the doctor now?

Jason nods and continues.

Jason: Soon. First, let me now ask you about your family and any health conditions you had in the past. Did any other close relatives have similar symptoms as the ones you have described?
Chun: Possibly. I cannot recall any specific cases.

Jason: Did you have any other medical conditions in the past that you took medication for?

Chun: No. Anyway, I was never a fan of modern medicine.

Jason: OK, Mrs Bowie. I will inform my GP about your case, and she will get back to you soon.

Chun: So I am not going to see the doctor today?

Jason: Dr Rogers is busy with other patients at the moment. She will call you in a short while to discuss your condition. If you wish, you can wait to see her, but it may take a while.

Chun nods and continues to wait for the doctor.

DISCUSS

1. What social issues could be identified through this consultation?
2. What does Jason suspect is a possible diagnosis?
3. How does Chun respond to some of Jason's comments?

FURTHER DEVELOPMENTS

Dr Jill Rogers asks Jason to brief her on Chun's condition in order that they may diagnose her or, at the very least, acquire a general understanding of the case. Due to the fact that Jason is undergoing training, Dr Rogers asks him to summarise the case, diagnose the patient (if he can on the basis of the available information), and justify his decision. Jason concludes that the patient has depression and she should be referred to a psychiatrist or clinical psychologist for proper assessment. Jason also highlights that the patient combines social characteristics which are associated with mental illness, such as socioeconomic background, gender, ethnicity, and age. Dr Rogers agrees and schedules a meeting with the patient to inform her accordingly.

DISCUSS

1. Why does Jason appear to be so sure about his diagnosis?
2. What does Jason mean by saying that age, gender, social class, poverty, and place of origin contribute to the development of depression?

SOCIAL CLASS AND MENTAL ILLNESS

Dr Jill: Jason, could you please outline the literature on the relationship between mental illness and social background? It would be useful to have this information to help us better support our diagnosis.

Jason: Yes, I would be happy to do that. It is a good opportunity for me to revise and remember the material I was taught.

Based on Chun's account, she appears to be experiencing financial difficulties. While Jason is right to highlight that there is evidence to suggest a relationship between social class and diseases in general, and mental health in particular, there are studies that have not established such a link.

In this section, I rely heavily on Rogers and Pilgrim's (2010) book, *A Sociology of Mental Health and Illness*, which summarises the findings from a series of studies, which show the relationship between mental health and social class. Rogers and Pilgrim cite an early study by Faris and Dunham from 1939 that revealed the relevance of economic background to mental illness in Chicago and found that people with schizophrenia and psychosis were more likely to come from the poor economic classes, more specifically from poor areas in the city. The researchers argued that the reason for this had to do with both poverty and poor social integration in these areas (see also Cockerham, 2011). The primary cause of these living conditions was chronic stress, which might have led to psychosis later in life. This early study indicated the role of social context and isolation in people's health status and was endorsed by Dunham who published a study in 1957.

Rogers and Pilgrim cited more recent studies of the association between social class and mental illness. More specifically, a later review of 21 studies from 1950 to 1980 by Dohrenwend et al. (1980), found a negative relationship between socioeconomic status and mental illness. That is, the lower the socioeconomic status, the higher the rates of mental illness. In 1988, Hudson further confirmed this relationship by reviewing studies from the 1980s. In the 1990s, Link et al. found that people who had an occupation with an increased sense of control and planning were more likely to be protected from depression. Detracting from the genealogy of mental illness, Weich and Lewis (1998) indicated that poverty and unemployment heightened depression but did not seem to contribute to the onset of the disorder. In 2001, Ritsher et al. published the findings from 756 interviews and one of the main findings indicated that depression was associated with a low level of education among the individual's parents.

Interestingly, Rogers and Pilgrim (2010) presented studies that did not support the link between social class and mental illness. For example, Clausen and Kohn's (1959) study of psychosis in Hagerstown found no relationship between depression and social isolation. Along similar lines, Weinberg, as well as Gerard and Houston, who published their works in 1960 and 1953, respectively, failed to establish a connection between social background and mental illness. Later studies by Srole et al. (1962) and Langner and Michael (1963) showed that psychotic symptoms in the United States were more common among lower-class individuals, while neurotic symptoms were more common among the middle class (this difference derived from over-controlling the ambition of middle-class children). Rogers and Pilgrim (2010, p. 52) explained that out of these contradictory findings two approaches have emerged. *First*, the 'drift hypothesis', which puts forward that patients with mental illness tend to live in socially disadvantaged areas or they cannot move upwards in the social hierarchy. In other words, it is the presence of mental illness that causes these people to have lower socioeconomic status. *Second*, the 'opportunity and stress' hypothesis points to the social circumstances that lead to stress, which in turn, results in mental disorders. Rogers and Pilgrim (2010) argue that there are studies that support both hypotheses, depending on the mental disorder. For example, Dohrenwend et al. (1992) found that depression in women had to do with socioeconomic background (opportunity and stress hypothesis); however, schizophrenia was connected to lower social class possession (the drift hypothesis). Wiggins et al. (2004) presented an even more complicated relationship between social class and mental illness by finding that minor mental disorders were associated with social class only when other social factors, such as unemployment, were at play. The two hypotheses that Rogers and Pilgrim have outlined reflect the two classical approaches to the negative relationship between social class and mental illness, which have derived from the questions: is it social class that makes people more susceptible to mental illness or are people who are predisposed to mental illness, biologically, more likely to be unable to move upwards in the social hierarchy? The first question is attached to the approach of 'social causation' (or materialist), whereas the second is to the approach of 'social selection' (see Chapter 6, 'Social Inequalities in Health', for a thorough explanation of these terms).

Hudson (2005) aimed to test these two hypotheses (social causation and social selection) empirically. He planned a longitudinal study in the Commonwealth of Massachusetts of people who had been hospitalised due to mental illness during the period 1994–2000. Hudson used the

2000 US Census, which represented the socioeconomic status of patients based on individual records of patients. The results revealed a strong negative correlation between mental illness and socioeconomic status and, more specifically, found that the correlation lay within the community and not across individuals, in the sense that it was not the same individuals who experienced mental illness. Hudson's main hypothesis was not merely to establish the relationship between mental illness and socioeconomic status, but to test whether socioeconomic status and the lack of family integrity led to mental illness. The study showed that socioeconomic status had a direct impact on mental illness, thereby supporting the theory of social causation, whereas no link with the social selection theory was established. Interestingly, the research findings above do not seem to have changed over the years. A 2016 report by the Mental Health Foundation in the UK showed that children and adults living in households with the lowest income were significantly more likely to have mental illness. Reiss et al. (2019) found similar results in their study among children and adolescents in Germany.

Jason completes his assignment and submits it to Dr Rogers to review.

Dr Jill: Thank you for your thorough account, Jason! Are there any other social factors that might play a role?

Jason: Yes, there are. Gender, age, and migration are also influential factors.

Dr Jill: Please tell me more about these factors.

GENDER AND MENTAL ILLNESS

Chun is a woman and, as Jason has already pointed out, women are more vulnerable to developing mental disorders. Why is this the case? Evidence from the relevant literature shows that women are more likely than men to report mental illnesses, but this does not necessarily mean that they are more vulnerable. It might mean that they are more likely to seek help and to communicate their mental condition to other people. Rogers and Pilgrim (2010) present research information that shows that women are more susceptible than men to chronic stress. This chronic stress results from the increased pressure exerted on women on account of their demanding social roles, which they are expected to perform successfully (i.e., mother, wife, and employee). Rogers and Pilgrim (2010, p. 71) refer to specific factors that have a negative impact on women's psychological state. *First,* there are various 'vulnerability factors' that relate to possible events in a woman's life, such as poor care after the loss of a mother at an early age, the lack of a relationship with a partner, the absence of employment, and having three or more children. *Second*, there are the 'provoking agents', which have to do with events in daily life, such as the loss of a loved one, divorce, or having a serious health condition. *Third*, the 'symptom-formation' factors refer to the psychological characteristics that nurture depression. These include low self-esteem, feeling discredited, and having been sexually or physically abused during childhood. Chun seems to have been provoked by specific agents in her life, which might have caused her psychological condition to develop. These include her husband dying in a car accident, her sons leaving the country, and her now living alone in the UK.

Other scholars either support Rogers and Pilgrim or point out other reasons for the gender difference that seems to exist in depression. More specifically, Afifi (2007) argued that adolescent girls were more likely than boys to suffer from depression and adult women developed depression and psychosis more often than men. Depression, according to Afifi, is a way to respond to stress. Interestingly, men appeared to respond to stress differently, by behaving antisocially and abusing alcohol. Afifi (2007, p. 387) stated that 'chronic strain, low mastery, and rumination' were more likely to be experienced by women than by men and might have resulted in prompting symptoms of depression. Reviewing the literature, Piccinelli and Wilkinson (2000) concurred that women were more likely than men to have depression and that there were specific reasons for this. *First*, women were more likely to have experienced anxiety during their adolescence, which manifested itself in depressive episodes later in life. *Second*, women were regarded as having a more devalued role in modern society, such as that of mother or homemaker. Interestingly, evidence from societies that still value these roles, such as the Mediterranean cultures, indicates that the relationship between depression and gender is weak. *Third*, evidence indicated that women experienced negative events in their life more intensely and, as a result, were more vulnerable to depression. Women interpreted their life events differently and were more likely to pay more attention to them and analyse their causes, whereas men were more likely to be engaged in physical activities, which helped focus their attention towards more pleasant activities.

A large-scale comparative study in 23 European countries by Van de Velde et al. (2010) supported some of the findings and explanations summarised above. The study relied on the European Social Survey (ESS), in which 36,752 people aged 18–75 participated. Interestingly, the study showed that depression rates were higher in Eastern European countries and lower in Northern and Western European countries. However, gender differences were not only observed in Eastern European countries but also in Southern European countries (contrary to Afifi's assumption about the Mediterranean countries). Traditionally, countries in these two areas of Europe considered men as the main breadwinners in the family, while, in reality, both men and women worked in order to support their families. However, these countries were in the process of transitioning from traditional to modern lifestyles, and many women found themselves in the labour market, thus performing multiple roles in society. With the exception of Bulgaria and Hungary, women were more likely than men to report depression. The protective factors, for both men and women, were found to be a better socioeconomic position and family status (i.e., marriage and cohabitation), while education seemed to protect women from falling into depression, possibly because women were likely to have lower salaries than men and, thus, relied on education in order to improve their quality of life. In support, Girgus and Yang (2015) stressed that depression was more prevalent among women and focused more on the importance of social stress, explaining that men and women were triggered by different stressors, and they employed different mechanisms to cope. Interestingly, although Albert (2015) also highlighted the gender difference in depression, he pointed out the impact of genetics and hormonal changes.

Coming back to our case, Chun serves as an example of a woman who has not received higher education and, as such, undertook various jobs throughout her working life; she did not have the opportunity to pursue a long-term career. However, she was well protected from mental illness for many years as a wife and mother, who found meaning through raising her children and taking care of her husband. These roles were lost when her husband died, her children grew up and left the country, and Chun was left with few financial resources and friends to socialise with. Her new social circumstances, drawing from the literature, seem to have placed Chun at a greater risk of developing depression. With the passing of time, Chun grew older; advanced age is also associated with increased rates of mental illness.

AGE AND MENTAL ILLNESS

More recent evidence shows that developing mental illness is a complicated matter and that there is no one factor at play, while different mental disorders are associated with different risks. Studies show that age is one factor that influences mental illness, which is more likely to be observed among younger people (Blackmore, 2019; Twenge et al., 2019). A large-scale meta-analysis of 192 studies and 708,561 participants by Solmi et al. (2021) found that globally the first mental disorder was likely to have happened before the age of 14 in about 30% of participants. Interestingly, the rate was 48.5% and 62.5% for individuals younger than 18 and 25, respectively. In addition, the meta-analysis revealed that the peak age was 14.5 and the median age was 18. These results strongly suggest that younger people are quite vulnerable in developing mental illness. The reasons vary and the mechanism of developing mental illness is not simple. Blackmore (2019) explained that the period before adulthood was the time for developmental changes psychologically, biologically, and socially. Blackmore carried on emphasising that the brain is changing rapidly during adolescence and such changes might cause younger individuals to be vulnerable to mental illness. Twenge et al.'s (2019) study showed that between 2008 and 2017, serious mental episodes increased among younger people (ages 18–25) and did not have to do so much with unemployment or substance abuse, because during the period of the study unemployment rates had decreased while drug use remained relatively stable. The authors pointed out the importance of much engagement with social media, cyberbullying, and lack of face-to-face interactions. In support, a rapid literature review by Racine et al. (2020) indicated an increase in depressive and anxiety symptoms during a period of social isolation and uncertainly due to the COVID-19 pandemic which might have caused younger people to experience fear of infection or losing a beloved one.

Interestingly, a meta-umbrella study by Arrango et al. (2021), which studied umbrella reviews (combination of systematic reviews and meta-analyses), mapped the risk factors for mental illness and found that different disorders were associated with different risks. For instance, widowhood, sexual dysfunction, physical abuse in childhood, job stress, and obesity were associated with depression. Past traumatic experiences and sexual abuse in childhood were linked with post-traumatic disorders. The authors also found that some risk factors were associated with many disorders. For example, adverse experiences in childhood were associated with borderline personality disorder, bipolar disorder, and schizophrenia spectrum disorders.

In addition to mental illness in childhood and adolescence, there is research evidence to suggest that older people may suffer from depression too. More specifically, the survey by Mann et al. (cited in Rogers and Pilgrim, 2010) in London showed that two-fifths of the residents of the city had depression. Surveys in Australia conducted by Snowden and Donnelly (cited in Rogers and Pilgrim, 2010) suggested that nearly one-third of elderly people were depressed; a study in Italy by Spagnoll (cited in Rogers and Pilgrim, 2010) revealed similar findings. Other studies did not show different results from the studies cited by Rogers and Pilgrim. Roberts et al. (1997) studied depression among 2,730 participants, aged 46 and older in 1994 and 1995, and found that depression rates went up from 1994 to 1995 among people who were older than 60. This rate was even higher among the participants who were older than 80. Stordal et al. (2001; 2003) analysed data from more than 60,000 subjects in Norway and found that depression rates increased in advanced age. Van't Veer-Tazelaar et al. (2008) identified a gap in the literature that underrepresented participants who were older than 75 years old. On this note, they studied 2,850 individuals from 2003 to 2006 in the Netherlands. They found that approximately one-third of the participants were depressed, significantly higher than their younger counterparts.

Rogers and Pilgrim (2010) outlined a series of reasons why older people were likely to have depression. *First*, older people who found themselves in nursing homes tended to be depressed largely due to being relatively inactive and as a result of the disruptive experience they went through as they moved from their home to a nursing home. *Second*, older people were more likely than younger people to suffer from chronic diseases which, as explained in Chapter 3, might be experienced as a 'biographical disruption' (Bury, 1982). *Third*, older people increasingly lose friends and relatives due to the biological event of death. *Fourth*, socioeconomic background when younger, or experience of social and economic deprivation, work as factors for increasing the rate of depression among the elderly. *Fifth*, the absence of supportive relationships seemed to be a fact that depressed older people. *Sixth*, abuse was another experience some older people may suffer from, and this places them at risk of developing depression.

MIGRATION AND MENTAL ILLNESS

Based on the literature, it seems that Chun possesses all the social characteristics that could potentially make someone susceptible to mental illness. Above, I have shown how socioeconomic background, gender, and age have placed Chun at risk of developing a mental illness. Another social characteristic that makes Chun even more vulnerable is the fact that she is a migrant. Research evidence indicates an association between migration and mental illness.

Bhugra and Jones (2001) outlined the stages of migration that might have a negative impact on the wellbeing of migrants. They started with individuals' decision to migrate, the pre-migration stage, and continued with migration and post-migration when individuals were subject to cultural shock. Individuals might take various routes, such as assimilation, acculturation, and deculturation. Bhugra and Jones (2001) summarised several studies of how the consequences of migration were associated with mental illness. More specifically, studies of schizophrenia in the UK during the 1980s and 1990s indicated that the prevalence of the mental illness was higher among migrants than local people, while similar trends were observed in the Netherlands. Studies revealed that African-Caribbean people living in the UK had the highest rates of schizophrenia, while Asian people did not appear to suffer more from the disease compared to the local population. Bhugra and Jones (2001) presented a series of hypotheses to account for these findings. *First*, migrants tended to have higher schizophrenia rates in their place of origin. This alluded to a biological predisposition towards schizophrenia; however, research evidence did not support this. *Second*, people with mental illness tended to migrate; again, this was not supported by the research. *Third*, migrants experienced chronic stress. Stress has been associated with schizophrenia; not in a direct way but through the interplay of other factors, such as social class, poverty, unemployment, and housing conditions. *Fourth*, migrants were more likely to be misdiagnosed. Such arguments were not supported since not all ethnic groups were more likely to have schizophrenia compared to the native population. As far as other mental illnesses were concerned, research studies cited by Bhugra and Jones (2001) showed that Indian and Pakistani migrants were more likely to report emotional disorders than White British, while Greek Cypriots had higher rates of anxiety compared to the British locals. Interestingly, Indian, Pakistani, Bangladeshi, Chinese, and Caribbean women living in the UK had lower anxiety rates. Bhugra and Jones (2001, p. 219) argued that what makes migrants more vulnerable was not migration per se but rather 'ethnic density'. In areas where the number of people from the same ethnic group was significant, rates of mental illness tended to drop, whereas in areas where the population was not large, as in the case of African-Caribbean people, the rate went up. It is in these well-integrated social contexts that people construct and reaffirm their social identity and have social support, which results in an improvement of their self-esteem. A later review of the literature by Bhugra (2004) revealed similar findings. See Chapter 8 for more details about ethnicity and health.

The case of African-Caribbean people was analysed more carefully by Sharpley et al. (2001). Drawing from research evidence, they ruled out misdiagnosis, tendency towards migration, prenatal or perinatal complications, use of cannabis, area of residence, and genetics as contributing factors towards schizophrenia. The authors did not reach safe conclusions as to why this might be the case, but they associated mental illness with the fact that hallucinations and paranoid ideas were more likely to be observed among African-Caribbeans and, thus, African-Caribbean people were more likely to be diagnosed. Further, the authors observed that African-Caribbean people tended to have socially disadvantaged backgrounds, such as being raised by single parents, living in poverty, and experiencing unemployment. Cockerham (2011) suggested that the inferior position of migrants in society leads to feelings of lower self-esteem and a subordinated self-image, which may place migrants at risk for mental illness.

Based on the information above, migration is a strong social factor which may cause people to be vulnerable to mental illness. The issue seems to be even more important nowadays with migration waves in many European countries. In the article 'The Mental-Health Crisis among Migrants', Abbott (2016) has highlighted the link between mental illness and migration. Meyer, Lasaster, and Tol's (2017) systematic review also showed an association between migration and mental illness. Interestingly, Hajak et al.'s (2021) systematic review found that the factors contributing to asylum seekers' mental illness are uncertainty about asylum status, shared accommodation, being away from family, poor integration, and discrimination.

From the literature above, it seems that Chun has been vulnerable to depression because of her low socioeconomic status, gender, age, and migration status in the sense that she lives alone. Having in mind the findings of Roberts et al. (1997) about the predictability of depression as age advances coupled with the lack of social networks in Chun's life (which will become more important and necessary for her at the time of chronic illness), Chun is placed at a higher risk for having chronic mental illness in the future.

FURTHER DEVELOPMENTS

Dr Jill: Thank you Jason, this is very helpful. I am now going to call Chun into my office to examine her and discuss our conclusion.
Chun enters Dr Rogers's office and takes a seat.

Dr Jill: Hello, Mrs Bowie. I am Dr Jill Rogers. Thank you for waiting to see me. How are you?

Chun [smiles]: Fine, thank you.

> *Dr Jill performs all necessary examinations and intends to inform Chun about the diagnosis.*

Chun: I told your medical student all that he wanted to know.

Dr Jill: Yes, I know. Jason gave me a very good overview of your symptoms, as well as your social, family, and past medical histories.

Chun: OK, can you please tell me what is wrong with me and how I can treat it?

Dr Jill: Well, examining everything together, the condition that is causing you to suffer from all the symptoms is depression. You will need to see a specialist in order to further investigate and confirm diagnosis.

Chun: What do you mean?

Dr Jill: I am sorry. Depression is a condition ... [*Chun interrupts Dr Rogers*].

Chun: I know what depression is. What do you mean I have depression?

> *Dr Jill Rogers and Jason look at each other.*

Dr Jill: Well, depression is a psychological disorder, which may develop as a result of the social environment and the everyday pressures people experience.

Chun: And how did you reach this conclusion? What have you relied on to come up with this diagnosis?

Dr Jill: Mrs Bowie, please calm down and allow me to explain the condition. You have said that you feel tired, dizzy, and that you experience pain throughout your body, correct?

Chun: Yes, that's right.

Dr Jill: You have also indicated that you cannot find any meaning in your life and that you feel sad.

Chun: No, I never said that. I just told Jason that I tend to stay home all the time. And I am not sad!

Dr Jill: Mrs Bowie, it is OK to feel that way, but you seem sad to me and staying at home all the time does not allow you to experience any social interactions, which is another factor that might have contributed to your depression.

Chun: You are not listening to me. I have always believed that Western medicine is not reliable and I tried natural remedies for many health conditions I had, but I could not find a solution for the symptoms I am experiencing now and that's why I decided to come here. Obviously, I was wrong. I am trying to tell you that something is wrong with my body, and you are trying to convince me that something is wrong with my mind. This is a wrong approach; if you want to make a proper diagnosis then listen to what I am telling you.

Dr Jill: Mrs Bowie, there is no diagnosis on the basis of the physical symptoms you have described, especially given that all of the medical tests you had are clear.

> *Chun does not say anything more and leaves the GP clinic disappointed and frustrated. Jason is upset by what has happened and Dr Jill Rogers assures him that it is common to experience difficult patients.*

Dr Jill: If her symptoms persist then Chun will most likely come back. In the meantime, could you research something for me? It will be a good learning opportunity for you as well.

Jason: Yes, of course. What do you have in mind, Doctor?

Dr Jill: Could you please explore the social sciences literature based on our experience here in order to see whether we have missed anything important or whether there is something we cannot easily see and understand. If we missed something, then we will approach Chun differently next time.

Jason: Yes. Do you suspect something in particular?

Dr Jill: Nothing specific. Chun sounded adamant about not suffering from depression even though she has all the symptoms. Perhaps it might have to do with cultural influences; she comes from China, right? Please look into it and let me know. You do not need to write a long report; one page would be fine.

DISCUSS

1. Why is there a difference between Chun and Dr Rogers's approach to the problem?
2. What should Jason be looking for in the social sciences literature?
3. Could people from China interpret their depressive symptoms differently than people in North America and Western Europe?

DEPRESSION IN CHINA

> *Jason reads the relevant literature and becomes excited when the information he finds sheds some light on Chun's experience and reaction. He prepares the following short report for Dr Rogers.*

Kleinman (2004, p. 951) argued that people from China expressed depression in physical symptoms, not psychologically; that is, they tended to express 'boredom, discomfort, feelings of inner pressure, and symptoms of pain, dizziness, and fatigue'. Kleinman explained that many Chinese migrants did not eagerly accept the Western diagnosis of depression, while clinicians in the West appear not to be acquainted with the way in which Chinese people express their depressive symptoms. As a result, depression among Chinese people was either underreported or undiagnosed. Ryder et al. (2008) conducted an empirical study of the ideas above by comparing 196 Chinese (in Changsha, China) and 123 Canadian (Toronto, Canada) patients. The authors wanted to know whether Chinese patients indeed tended to report more somatic symptoms. A Structured Clinical Interview for Diagnostic and Statistical Manual of Mental Disorders (DSM-IV), Axis I, Patient Version was used to collect data. Interestingly, the results showed that Canadian participants reported more psychological symptoms than their Chinese counterparts. Although depression is China is rising (Huang et al., 2019), possibly because it is now more likely to be reported and diagnosed, recent evidence suggests that people from China, especially from rural areas, are still very likely to understand depression differently than how it is understood in other Western societies. More specifically, Qiu et al. (2018) used a vignette and asked 416 women to reflect on it. The results indicated that 66.6% of their participants thought that the person in the vignette had something wrong with their health, 54.3% referred to non-specific psychiatric diseases, 28.2% referred to physical diseases, and only 2.9% used a specific psychiatric disease name. As intervention, participants suggested seeing a doctor, solving the problem on their own, or approaching family members and friends. There were no specific suggestions for visiting a psychologist or a psychiatrist. Echoing Qui et al.'s findings, Huang et al. (2016) highlighted that many people in China did not seek treatment for psychological disorders. Shi et al.'s (2020) study revealed that the main barriers among Chinese people for not seeking help for psychological symptoms were self-reliance, using alternative sources, low perceived need, lack of affordability, negative attitude, stigma, family objection, poor experience with seeking help, limited knowledge about mental illness, fear of burdening the family, and preferred not telling. Interestingly, Evans-Lacko et al.'s (2012) study of public views and self-stigma in 14 countries showed that in countries where stigma was not as strong a barrier, higher rates of seeking help were observed.

Zhang (1995, pp. 228–9) described three main reasons why people from China tended not to describe depression in psychological terms.

First, traditional Chinese medicine did not use depression as a label or classification to account for any symptoms that would be considered as depression in the West. Instead, traditional Chinese medicine would attribute depression to too much anger, thinking, and worrying, and would diagnose someone as *shen-kui*, which meant that the symptoms came from a deficiency in the kidney functions and control over the cerebrum. Traditional Chinese medicine also diagnosed someone as *xie-ping*, which referred to a sickness coming from the devil. *Second*, Chinese people tended to prefer the diagnosis of neurasthenia, which meant 'neurological weakness' and pertained to dizziness, insomnia, reduced appetite, weakness, and so forth, thereby rejecting the label of depression due to the political connotations it carried. More specifically, during the Chinese Revolution the Maoists challenged all mental illnesses and labelled them as undesired 'political thinking' (see also Kleinman, 1988). *Third*, the Chinese preferred using the term neurasthenia because it was socially acceptable to describe their symptoms in bodily or physical terms rather than in physiological ones. Also, in China, people were not encouraged to seek help for any psychological conditions, but they were encouraged to do so when they experienced physical discomfort. Interestingly, Zhang (1995, p. 230) went on to argue that 'emotion in traditional Chinese literature is portrayed subtly and indirectly via body movements, dress, environmental description and allusive language, but not by direct verbal expression'.

Zhang (1995) suggested a few ways for improving consultation with Chinese patients. *First*, clinicians needed to be aware of cultural beliefs about health and cultural influences on people's understanding of health. *Second*, the clinician could utilise the label of neurasthenia and terms that traditional Chinese medicine uses, such as anger, thinking, and worrying, and ask questions that pertain to actions rather than feelings. *Third*, the clinician might ask the patient to bring objects they feel comfortable with to the consultation sessions, and thus have them express their emotions through these objects. In this way, the objects could work as mediators and patients would feel more comfortable talking about their emotions in this indirect way.

DISCUSS

How does this information explain Chun's attitudes and reaction?

FURTHER DEVELOPMENTS

Jason submitted his report to Dr Rogers who, in turn, embraced the information gleaned from the literature, which helped to explain Chun's reaction.

Dr Jill: This is very helpful information, Jason! Chun's reaction makes sense now and I wish I had known this scientific information before consulting with her. She may not return to us, but we can definitely use this information for any future patients. Perhaps it is good to first have an introductory consultation to gauge the patient's perceptions and cultural background, explore the literature a bit if needed and then proceed with history-taking.

Jason: It might be a good idea to organise a training session here in cultural competence for all the GPs and nurses. We could invite our medical sociologist to deliver the training.

Dr Jill: That's a brilliant idea! I am sure it will significantly aid us in improving our communication skills with patients and, subsequently, with the communication and explanation of future medical diagnoses. In Chun's case, it seems that we made a lot of assumptions, and cultural competence training would help us to provide the best possible care to diverse patients.

REFERENCES

Abbott A. The mental-health crisis among migrants. *Nature.* 2016; 538(7624): 158–60. https://doi.org/10.1038/538158a.

Afifi M. Gender differences in mental health. *Singapore Med J.* 2007; 48(5): 385–91.

Albert PR. Why is depression more prevalent in women? *J Psychiatry Neurosci.* 2015; 40(4): 219.

Arango C, Dragioti E, Solmi M, Cortese S, Domschke K, Murray RM, ... Fusar-Poli P. Risk and protective factors for mental disorders beyond genetics: An evidence-based atlas. *World Psychiatry.* 2021; 20(3): 417–36.

Bhugra D. Migration and mental health. *Acta Psychiatr Scand.* 2004; 109(4): 243–58.

Bhugra D, Jones P. Migration and mental illness. *Adv Psychiatr Treat.* 2001; 7(3): 216–23.

Blakemore SJ. Adolescence and mental health. *Lancet.* 2019; 393(10185): 2030–1.

Bury M. Chronic illness as biographical disruption. *Sociol Health Illn.* 1982; 4(2): 167–82.

Clausen JA, Kohn ML. Relation of schizophrenia to the social structure of a small city. In: Pasamanick B, editor. *Epidemiology of Mental Disorder.*

Washington, DC: American Association for the Advancement of Science; 1959, pp. 69–94.

Cockerham WC. *Sociology of Mental Disorder.* 8th ed. Boston, MA: Prentice Hall; 2011.

Dohrenwend BP, Dohrenwend BS, Gould MS, Wunsch Hitzig RA, Link B, Neugebauer R. *Mental Illness in the United States: Epi-Demiological Estimates.* New York: Praeger; 1980.

Dohrenwend BP, Levav I, Shrout PE, Schwartz S, Naveh G, Link BG, Skodol AE, Stueve A. Socioeconomic status and psychiatric disorders: The causation-selection issue. *Science.* 1992; 255(5047): 946–52.

Dunham HW. Methodology of sociological investigations of mental disorders. *Int J Soc Psychiatry.* 1957; 3(1): 7–17.

Evans-Lacko S, Brohan E, Mojtabai R, Thornicroft G. Association between public views of mental illness and self-stigma among individuals with mental illness in 14 European countries. *Psychol Med.* 2012; 42(8): 1741–52.

Faris REL, Dunham HW. *Mental Disorders in Urban Areas: An Ecological Study of Schizophrenia and Other Psychoses.* Oxford: University of Chicago Press; 1939.

Gerard DL, Houston LG. Family setting and the social ecology of schizophrenia. *Psychiatr Q.* 1953; 27(1): 90–101.

Girgus JS, Yang K. Gender and depression. *Curr Opin Psychol.* 2015; 4: 53–60.

Hajak VL, Sardana S, Verdeli H, Grimm S. A systematic review of factors affecting mental health and well-being of asylum seekers and refugees in Germany. *Front Psychiatry.* 2021; 12: 315.

Huang Y, Liu Z, Wang H., Guan X, Chen H, Ma C, … Tan L. The China mental health survey (CMHS): I. background, aims and measures. *Soc Psychiatry Psychiatr Epidemiol.* 2016; 51(11): 1559–69.

Huang Y, Wang YU, Wang H, Liu Z, Yu X, Yan J, … Wu Y. Prevalence of mental disorders in China: A cross-sectional epidemiological study. *Lancet Psychiatry.* 2019; 6(3): 211–24.

Hudson CG. Socioeconomic status and mental illness: Implications of the research for policy and practice. *J Sociol Soc Welf.* 1988; 15(1): 27–54.

Hudson CG. Socioeconomic status and mental illness: Tests of the social causation and selection hypotheses. *Am J Orthopsychiatr.* 2005; 75(1): 3–18.

Kleinman A. *Rethinking Psychiatry.* New York: Free Press; 1988.

Kleinman A. Culture and depression. *N Engl J Med.* 2004; 351(10): 951–3.

Langner TS, Michael ST. *Life Stress and Mental Health* (Midtown Manhattan Study v. 2). New York: Free Press of Glencoe; 1963.

Link BG, Lennon MC, Dohrenwend BP. Socioeconomic status and depression: The role of occupations involving direction, control and planning. *Am J Sociol.* 1993; 98(6): 1351–87.

Mental Health Foundation. *Fundamental Facts about Mental Health 2016.* London: Mental Health Foundation; 2016.

Meyer SR, Lasater M, Tol WA. Migration and mental health in low-and middle-income countries: A systematic review. *Psychiatry.* 2017; 80(4): 374–81.

Piccinelli M, Wilkinson G. Gender differences in depression: Critical review. *Br J Psychiatry.* 2000; 177(6): 486–92.

Racine N, Cooke JE, Eirich R, Korczak DJ, McArthur B, Madigan S. Child and adolescent mental illness during COVID-19: A rapid review. *Psychiatry Res.* 2020; 292: 113307.

Reiss F, Meyrose AK, Otto C, Lampert T, Klasen F, Ravens-Sieberer U. Socioeconomic status, stressful life situations and mental health problems in children and adolescents: Results of the German BELLA cohort-study. *PLOS ONE.* 2019; 14(3): e0213700.

Ritsher JE, Warner V, Johnson JG, Dohrenwend BP. Inter-generational longitudinal study of social class and depression: A test of social causation and social selection models. *Br J Psychiatry Suppl.* 2001; 40: s84–90.

Qiu P, Caine ED, Hou F, Cerulli C, Wittink MN. Depression as seen through the eyes of rural Chinese women: Implications for help-seeking and the future of mental health care in China. *J. Affect. Disord.* 2018; 227: 38–47.

Roberts RE, Kaplan GA, Shema SJ, Strawbridge WJ. Does growing old increase the risk for depression? *Am J Psychiatry.* 1997; 154(10): 1384–90.

Rogers A, Pilgrim D. *A Sociology of Mental Health and Illness.* 4th ed. Glasgow: Open University Press; 2010.

Ryder AG, Yang J, Zhu X, Yao S, Yi J, Heine SJ, Bagby RM. The cultural shaping of depression: Somatic symptoms in China, psychological symptoms in North America? *J Abnorm Psychol.* 2008; 117(2): 300–13.

Sharpley MS, Hutchinson G, McKenzie K, Murray RM. Understanding the excess of psychosis among the African-Caribbean population in England: Review of current hypotheses. *Br J Psychiatry* 2001; 178(40): 560–8.

Shi W, Shen Z, Wang S, Hall BJ. Barriers to professional mental health help-seeking among Chinese adults: A systematic review. *Front Psychiatry.* 2020; 11: 442.

Solmi M, Radua J, Olivola M, Croce E, Soardo L, de Pablo GS, ... Fusar-Poli P. Age at onset of mental disorders worldwide: Large-scale meta-analysis of 192 epidemiological studies. *Mol Psychiatry.* 2021; 27(1): 1–15.

Srole L, Langner TS, Michael ST. *Mental Health in the Metropolis.* (Midtown Manhattan Study v. 1). New York: McGraw-Hill; 1962.

Stordal E, Kruger BM, Dahl NH, Krüger Ø, Mykletun A, Dahl AA. Depression in relation to age and gender in the general population: The Nord-Trøndelag Health Study (HUNT). *Acta Psychiatr Scand.* 2001; 104: 201–16.

Stordal E, Mykletum A, Dahl AA. The association between age and depression in the general population: A multivariate examination. *Acta Psychiatr Scand.* 2003; 107(2): 132–41.

Twenge JM, Cooper AB, Joiner TE, Duffy ME, Binau SG. Age, period, and cohort trends in mood disorder indicators and suicide-related outcomes in a nationally representative dataset, 2005–2017. *J Abnorm Psychol.* 2019; 128(3): 185.

Van de Velde S, Bracke P, Levecque K. Gender differences in depression in 23 European countries. Cross-national variation in the gender gap in depression. *Soc Sci Med.* 2010; 71(2): 305–13.

van't Veer-Tazelaar PJ, van Marwijk HW, Jansen AP, Rijmen F, Kostense PJ, van Oppen P, van Hout HP, Stalman WA, Beekman AT. Depression in old age (75+), the PIKO Study. *J Affect Disord* 2008; 106(3): 295–9.

Weich S, Lewis G. Poverty, unemployment, and common mental disorders: Population based cohort study. *BMJ.* 1998; 317(7151): 115–19.

Weinberg SK. Social psychological aspects of schizophrenia. In: Appleby L, Scher JM, Comming J, editors. *Chronic Schizophrenia.* pp. 68–88. Glencoe, IL: Free Press; 1960.

Wiggins RD, Schofield P, Sacker A, Head J, Bartley M. Social position and minor psychiatric morbidity over time in the British Household Panel survey 1991–1998. *J Epidemiol Community Health.* 2004; 58(9): 779–87.

Zhang D. Depression and culture: A Chinese perspective. *Can J Counsell.* 1995; 29(3): 227–33.

CHAPTER 6

Social inequalities in health

··

ABSTRACT

This chapter presents Mr George Winters's heart attack experience and the preconceptions that exist about the social distribution of diseases and how this is contrary to existing sociological literature, which shows that people from lower socioeconomic classes have higher morbidity and mortality rates. Ultimately, George's GP uses this information to better inform the patient and convince him to change certain aspects of his lifestyle, which are subject to cultural influences. This chapter aims to help healthcare students and practitioners to better understand inequalities in health, their impact on patients' lives and understanding of health, and to provide guidance in working more effectively with diversity.

LEARNING OBJECTIVES

- Identify the relationship between social class and health.
- Explain the role of education and individual behaviour in health and illness.
- Critically evaluate the materialist and behavioural models of explaining the relationship between social class and health.
- Describe life-course and psychosocial models to explain the relationship between social class and health.

DOI: 10.1201/9781003256687-7

- Define global health and outline key research areas.
- Explain structural competence and its usefulness in providing healthcare.

Note: Think about or discuss the questions that are in the boxes before you continue reading through the chapter.

SCENARIO

Mr George Winters is rushed to the emergency unit of a hospital near his house. He complained of severe chest pain and then fell unconscious. At the emergency unit, his wife could barely speak from shock, but she did mention that he had said something about experiencing chest pains before he passed out. Both the nurses and the doctors noted this as a crucial cue, which indicated a possible heart attack. Mr Winters was lucky enough to survive such an episode and, following a series of examinations, the diagnosis was indeed a heart attack. His wife provided the attending doctor with a brief medical, family, and social history of her husband. The doctor waited for Mr Winters to wake up and feel strong enough to talk, in order to get first-hand information about his history. The doctor managed to speak to his patient two days after the incident. Dr Ian Roberts asked about past medical, family, and medication history. He also found out that Mr Winters is married with three daughters, has a low-paid unskilled manual job, finished high school, smokes 25 cigarettes a day, drinks five small beers a day, and two to three drinks of heavier alcohol each week.

DISCUSS

1. What social aspects has Dr Ian Roberts explored?
2. How do social aspects or factors influence people's health?

FURTHER DEVELOPMENTS

George's condition improves, and after five days in the intensive care unit he is moved to a bigger room with other patients. The bed next to him is occupied by a patient, Matt Locker, who has also had a heart attack. Matt, a 55-year-old carpenter, is married with two children.

George: Hi. How long have you been here? Today is my fifth day. I'm here because I had a heart attack.

Matt: Me too; I've been here for six days.

George: I just cannot believe that I've had a heart attack at the age of 50. It just seems too young! I suppose this disease can affect anyone.

Matt: What do you mean?

George: Well, I mean that all people get sick, regardless of their age or background.

Matt: Don't be so sure about that. I know someone who is 70 years old, and he never gets sick. He is well off so he can visit the best doctors. I also think he has a more relaxing life and can afford to eat healthy food, which is usually quite expensive.

George: So you think that money can make such a difference to one's health?

Matt: I do.

George: Yes, but even rich people become ill and die like the rest of us.

Matt: Yes, but perhaps they live longer than others and enjoy a better quality of life.

A nurse, Annette Kelly, is attending to another patient nearby and overhears the conversation between George and Matt.

Annette: You are right. There is research evidence, largely from the field of sociology, which supports your view.

George: What research evidence?

Annette: Well, as nursing students, we attended several medical sociology lectures, which discussed the social aspects of health. One of these aspects is what sociologists call 'inequalities in health', and the relevant research shows that people from lower socioeconomic backgrounds have higher mortality and morbidity rates – they are more likely to get sick and suffer from chronic conditions than people who are better off financially.

George: Really? Why is this the case? Does money really make a difference?

Annette: The issue is quite complex and has to do with chronic stress, differences in lifestyle, as well as different ways of interpreting symptoms.

George: Well, what can we do about this? We certainly cannot become rich in order to live longer.

Annette: Probably not, but you could follow a healthier lifestyle.

DISCUSS

1. Is Nurse Annette Kelly correct to point out the role of social class in health?
2. What is the relationship between social class, education, and health?
3. What is the role of individual behaviour in health and illness?
4. Are there other factors that play a role, such as personality traits or stress?

SOCIOECONOMIC BACKGROUND AND HEALTH

Nurse Annette Kelly's recollection of the medical sociology she was taught at nursing school is correct. George is intrigued and wants to learn more about the subject.

George: Mrs Kelly, could you please tell me more about it; it sounds interesting but also somewhat frightening.

Annette presents the following information to both George and Matt.

Systematic research on the relationship between socioeconomic status and health dates back to the 1970s and has been conducted in the United States and Britain, as well as in other countries, such as Japan and the Netherlands. The general finding, which seems to be consistent across most studies, is that lower socioeconomic background is associated with higher mortality and morbidity rates. Interestingly, other factors such as education and lifestyle play a role; the literature shows that the impact of social factors, more specifically socioeconomic background, is more complex than it seems.

The study by Kitagawa and Hauser (1973) was among the first attempts to explore the relationship between social status and health. They drew information from two different sources of data. *First*, the 1960 Matched Records Study, which recorded the education background and income of individuals who died between May and August 1960 in the United States. *Second*, the Chicago Area Study, which stratified people living in the Chicago area by socioeconomic status; the study linked that status with mortality rates. Kitagawa and Hauser's findings were striking. The first set of data revealed that the lower the education level, the higher the mortality rates. A similar relationship was observed between household income and mortality. Interestingly, a closer analysis showed a strong relationship between a low level of education and mortality due to heart attack. Kitagawa and Hauser found that income did not interact with education in order to produce specific outcomes; rather, they worked independently. On this note, an explanation for the role of education was that schooling urged people to adopt healthier lifestyles. The second set of data was used to compare social class with mortality. Along the lines of the Matched Records Study, Kitagawa and Hauser found that lower social classes were associated with increased rates of mortality. Other studies such as that by Silver (1972) and Feldman et al. (1989) presented similar results.

One of the most popular publications in the area of social inequalities in health is the Black Report. The Black Report was supervised by Sir Douglas Black (Townsend and Davidson, 1990). Black and his research team classified the British population in six social classes, largely based on the occupation of the household's head. These six classes were class I: professional; class II: intermediate; class IIIN: skilled, non-manual; class IIIM: skilled, manual; class IV: partly skilled; and class V: unskilled. The team used the census to measure the number of people under each occupation/social class and then relied on death certificates to allocate deaths to each of the predefined occupations. In this case study, George would be classified under class V. Could belonging to this social class play a role in having a heart attack later in life? According to the Black Report, the answer would be yes. The results showed a steady increase in mortality rates, among both men and women, as social status moved from class I to class V.

The Black Report was controversial due to its methodological limitations; however, subsequent studies, which tried to overcome its limitations, indicated similar findings. For example, Bury (1997) clarified that studies that used data taken from the period following that examined by the Black Report showed that mortality rates of individuals who were classified as class V worsened. Data obtained during the 1990s, which was based on the same classification model, did not show any changes in mortality rates across the classes (Bartley and Blane, 2008). Whitehead's *The Health Divide* (Whitehead, 1990) presented results that were consistent with the findings described above, while Marmot and McDowall (1986), who used the same data as the Black Report but classified people only as manual and non-manual, found striking inequalities between the two groups in relation to heart disease and lung cancer.

The data presented in England and Wales each decade show interesting findings in terms of the causes of death, which also offer an indication of the types of diseases and morbidity distributed across the social classes (Bartley and Blane, 2008). For example, people from classes IV and V are more likely to die from heart diseases, lung cancer, and respiratory disease. Along similar lines, Blaxter (2010) argued that people from lower social classes are more likely to report suffering from chronic illness than individuals from the higher classes. In the 2000s, similar reports in the UK (cited in Russell, 2009) continued to show that mortality rates among people from class V were significantly higher than those among people from class I and that manual class members were more likely than non-manual class members to die from a heart attack.

Marmot's work has been highly influential in understanding the social determinants of health and how policy should be shaped accordingly. In his 2017 article 'The Health Gap', Marmot explained that the 'social gradient' (a term describing that disadvantageous socioeconomic position is linked with ill health; Donkin, 2014) was present and social inequalities in health still persisted even though the life expectancy has improved. Marmot clarified that this is not a case of the poor who are ill in comparison with the rich who are not. This is about the social gradient being present across the board, which means that all are affected. More specifically, even those who are near the top of the socioeconomic ladder are more affected than those at the top. Marmot (2020) carried on explaining that poorer healthy-life expectancy also relates to poorer socioeconomic background. Similar results have been found by Enroth and Fors (2021) and Hu et al. (2021).

George: I still do not understand. Does all this mean that, because I am not well off, I will die sooner that a man who is rich?

Annette: Not exactly. It means that, statistically speaking, you are more likely to pass away sooner than someone who has more money than you. However, you, yourself, might outlive many individuals who are better off than you.

George: Still, according to the literature, I am more vulnerable than them. It's like comparing heavy smokers to non-smokers?

Annette: Yes, more or less.

George: Is this true only in the US and the UK? If yes, perhaps I should move away from this country! [*Laughs*]

Interestingly, such studies have not only been confined to the United States and the United Kingdom. Kunst et al. (1990) studied health inequalities in the Netherlands. They noted that education and income were negatively associated with mortality. In Japan, Araki and Murata (1986) found that lower income was correlated with increased mortality; higher education was correlated with decreased mortality only among women. In Spain, women aged 22 to 44 years old from lower income social classes were more likely than women from higher income classes to have chronic illnesses, while in Poland, the higher the education level, the lower the mortality rate (Bartley and Blane, 2008). More recent studies have confirmed this. For example, Case and Deaton (2015) compared different countries in Europe and found that the bigger the gap in social gradient (e.g., education), the bigger is the difference in life expectancy.

George has raised a critical question about the possibility of getting sick because he comes from a working-class background. Morbidity is certainly more difficult to measure. Russell (2009) explained that manual workers were more likely to seek medical help compared to non-manual workers, but this did not necessarily mean that they were more likely to fall ill. Along similar lines, manual workers were more likely than non-manual workers to report experiences of chronic illness. Again, this did not necessarily indicate higher rates of morbidity – and could be attributed to different ways and levels of self-reporting health issues. Taylor and Field (2007) presented national statistics that showed that people in higher managerial positions were more likely to report good health than those in routine occupations or those who were never in the labour force and were unemployed. Moreover, people who worked on a full-time basis were more likely to describe their health as good compared to individuals who worked part time.

George: That's very disappointing. It sounds as though I am being punished because I am poor and I did not have the chance to pursue my higher education or, rather, I was not interested in higher education.

Annette: What do you mean by that?

George: You see, I grew up believing that God looked out for the poor people; that He is on our side and protects us. Now, I find out that the poor are dying younger and that they become ill more often than people from the higher social classes. It is purely injustice.

Annette: George, God has nothing to do with the matter. It actually relates more to human beings, their lifestyles, and to societies in general.

George: I would appreciate it if you could explain this to me in more detail.

WHY ARE DIFFERENCES IN MORTALITY AND MORBIDITY RATES OBSERVED?

The majority of studies that examine the relationship between socioeconomic status and health seem to reveal a negative association between socioeconomic status and mortality and morbidity. The data usually imply that there is a causal relationship. That is, social background causes, or at least influences mortality and morbidity. However, a correlation between two variables does not always indicate a causal relationship. This is the case with social class and health. Is it social class that makes the difference or individual behaviour? To answer this question, two main approaches have been developed and tested. These are: materialist (or social causation) and behavioural (Bartley et al., 1998).

The materialist approach focuses on people's access to resources such as housing, work, healthy environments, and healthcare. The behavioural approach pays attention to the individual and how the individual behaves in society with regards to habits or behaviours such as diet, smoking, physical exercise, drug use and abuse, as well as comprehension and utilisation of healthcare information. Research supports both approaches, and in many cases they seem to impact health together. Generally, studies show that resources, smoking, and biological factors play an important role in people's health. Interestingly, smoking has been proven to be associated with early mortality. Moreover, heavy smoking is more likely to be observed among people from the lower socioeconomic classes. Feldman et al. (1989) studied the relationship between smoking and mortality and found that mortality rates among heavy smokers were twice as high as those among non-smokers. However, smoking may interrelate with other behaviours, which are also more common among people from lower socioeconomic classes, such as stress and alcohol abuse. There is a critical question here: why are people from lower socioeconomic classes more likely to smoke? Layte and Whelan (2009) cited studies mainly from the 1990s to point out that working-class people were more likely to lack knowledge of the risks of smoking and that they adopted a more fatalistic approach to health and disease. Interestingly, Layte and Whelan's study indicated that lower education was associated with higher smoking prevalence and that the most influential factor was the experiences of social deprivation that working people went through. In other words, smoking is a coping mechanism for psychosocial stress. Marmot (2017) has already highlighted the importance of research findings showing that obesity, smoking, and heavy drinking are associated with lower socioeconomic status. Reasons vary from coping with stress, perceived lost control in daily life, lack of information, lost purpose, and lack of opportunities (Action on Smoking and Health, 2019).

Another factor that relates to social class, which has been associated with ill health, is the access and utilisation of healthcare services. Feinstein (1993, p. 312) outlined four main areas of utilisation, namely 'preventive care', 'diagnosis and entry into the healthcare system', 'treatment efficacy', and 'follow-up and readmission'. Feinstein presented examples with the support of research that showed the levels of utilisation by social classes in all these areas. More specifically, women from lower socioeconomic classes were less likely to get screened for breast or cervical cancer. Furthermore, diagnosis and hospitalisation, among people from lower socioeconomic statuses, occurred at later stages in the course of a disease. People from lower social classes also tended to have difficulties utilising and understanding healthcare services efficiently or they avoided exploring further options. Finally, patients from lower social classes had higher mortality rates, possibly due to the lack of knowledge about possible recurrences or relapses and the need for rehospitalisation.

Interestingly, many scholars have searched for other reasons to explain the differences between social groups as described above. That is, the results may be an artefact, meaning that there may be statistical products that they do not account for the complex social reality and the rapid changes that occur from one historical period to another (Bartley et al., 1998). Other scholars (see Bartley and Blane, 2008) point out that correlation does not equate with causation, an approach that has been called 'social selection'. According to the social selection approach, people who are likely to get sick, or are more vulnerable to diseases, tend to possess a lower position in society – what has also been called the 'drift hypothesis' for mental illness (see Rogers and Pilgrim, 2010, p. 52). Though both the artefact and the social selection approaches have their merits and validity, research data seems to largely support a combination of materialist and behavioural explanations, though research places more emphasis on the materialist approach. For example, Bartley and Blane (2008) argued that health behaviours explained only 30% of the differences in people's health and that, despite the observation that life expectancy has increased, health inequalities have remained relatively stable. Additionally, life expectancy has increased at a time when individuals have access to improved material resources, a fact that supports the materialist explanation.

Apart from the materialist and behavioural explanation, two more models have gained considerable attention. The first is the life-course model that aimed at connecting various influential factors. More specifically, Van de Mheen et al. (1998, p. 193) offered an alternative approach to conceptualise the mechanisms involved in the production of health inequalities and came up with three processes. The *first* has to do with the role of 'childhood socioeconomic conditions' and how these have influenced social class status in adulthood. This was a valid link to make in the sense that the childhood socioeconomic conditions experienced may have restricted a person's opportunities to move upwards along the social class hierarchy. Also, such childhood background might have affected opportunities for education and well-paying jobs. The *second* process links health conditions in childhood with health inequalities in adulthood. The *third* process relates to 'health selection' in adulthood and the question of whether socioeconomic background led to ill health or whether ill health kept people in the lower social classes. The life-course model placed personality, culture, and health behaviour at the centre of an individual's course. Personality, culture, and health behaviour were considered to be influenced by socioeconomic background and childhood health, which in turn impacted an individual's socioeconomic status and health in adulthood.

Van de Mheen et al. (1998, p. 196) tested their model empirically by using data from the Longitudinal Study of Socioeconomic Health Differences (LS-SEHD) in the Netherlands, and the findings were revealing. The results for the first process showed that individuals who grew up with a lower socioeconomic background were more at risk of developing ill health in adulthood. Interestingly, those who had experienced a lower socioeconomic background during both childhood and adulthood presented the highest risk. Socioeconomic status in childhood was also found to have an impact on possessing a neurotic personality later in life. Moreover, children with a lower socioeconomic background tended to be preoccupied with their local community and less likely to be future oriented. This might have influenced their health beliefs and behaviour in terms of seeking help and understanding medical information and processes. Interestingly, the authors found that the relationship between childhood socioeconomic status and health in adulthood was more likely to be explained by personality and cultural factors (50%) rather than by behaviour (10%). The results for the second process indicated that health conditions in childhood increased the risk of reporting 'less-than-good general health' by 5–10%. For the process of 'health selection', the authors did not find that health problems had an impact on people's social status.

The second model is the psychosocial model. Elstad (1998) argued that the models outlined above were insufficient, in the sense that they overlooked certain psychological dimensions and, thus, he analysed a psychosocial perspective to explain the inequalities in health. This model combined three approaches, namely the stress approach, the self-efficacy approach, and the social cohesion approach. The stress approach highlighted the importance of experienced stress in modern societies and showed that people from lower socioeconomic classes were more likely to experience stress compared to people from higher socioeconomic classes. The second approach focused on the role of the person's ability and their sense of having control and power over their life and in everyday tasks. Van de Mheen (1998) presented that the external locus of control (basically, low self-efficacy) was stronger among people from lower socioeconomic backgrounds. The third approach was based on the notion of relative poverty. That is, people were poor, not in absolute terms (lack of food, clothing, and housing) but in terms of how poor the other members of a given society were (the European Union considers individuals earning 60% below the median income as living in relative poverty). Living under conditions of relative poverty, poorer people were likely to feel disadvantaged and, as a result, feelings of social disintegration and stress might have accrued.

The psychosocial model seems to be applicable not only to people from lower socioeconomic backgrounds but also to people who have experienced forced migration. More specifically, Loizos and Constantinou (2007) found differences between refugees and non-refugees on the island of Cyprus when it came to heart disease; however, the difference was statistically significant only within a 10% margin of error. Loizos and Constantinou concluded that refugees in Cyprus did not experience the same amount of chronic stress as refugees who migrated from Eastern European countries after the World War II. This was attributed to the fact that they had not experienced significant cultural shock since they did not have to learn a new language; having fled from the northern part of Cyprus to the south, they found jobs in a relatively short period of time after being dislocated and, consequently, placed attainable cultural goals (e.g., to educate and marry off their children), which helped them regain meaning in life and oriented them to the future.

Marmot (2005), in a very important article, 'The Social Determinants of Health Inequalities', compared data from different countries, as well as within countries, and concluded that social factors, such as poverty and socioeconomic status per se, could not account for the differences observed. More specifically, Marmot presented data that showed that in Sierra Leone life expectancy was 34 years, compared to Japan, where this was almost 82 years. The mortality number per 1,000 children under five years old was shrinking across countries: 316 in Sierra Leone, 3 in Iceland, 4 in Finland, and 5 in Japan. While child mortality rates in Western countries have gone down, in countries such as Zimbabwe and Iraq, child mortality has increased by 43% and 75%, respectively. Comparing the rates within countries indicated that inequalities were observed between different social groups. In Indonesia, India, Brazil, and Kenya, the comparison between groups with different incomes (ranging from the five poorest groups to the five richest groups) showed that mortality rates among children younger than five years old was about three times higher among poor families. Mortality rates in the adult population followed a similar pattern, either across countries or within countries.

Marmot focused on Australian Aborigines and Torres Strait Islanders who had life expectancy rates much lower (56.3 years for men and 62.8 for women) than the general Australian life expectancy. This was neither due to high infant mortality nor to infectious diseases but, rather, due to 'non-communicable disease and injury'. The main causes of death among Australian Aborigines and Torres Strait Islanders were cardiovascular, cancer, endocrine, nutritional and metabolic diseases, respiratory and digestive diseases, and violent deaths. Marmot did not deny the importance of poverty, material deprivation, and unhealthy behaviour, such as smoking, drinking, and diet, but pointed out that particular attention should be paid to what caused these factors, which, in turn, could potentially lead to higher mortality rates. Based on gross national product per person, countries like Greece, Costa Rica, and Cuba were considered poor countries; however, they boasted a life expectancy as high as those found in rich countries. On this note, Marmot stressed the need to focus on the social determinants approach and understand how other factors play a role in people's health. Poverty might be responsible for ill health in sub-Saharan Africa, but it did not seem to be the main or only cause for the lower life expectancy rates among the Australian Aborigines and Torres Strait Islanders. Other social factors, such as the conditions in which people live and work, and how people respond to these conditions, are important clues to take into consideration in order to sufficiently understand health inequalities. The World Health Organization (Wilkinson and Marmot, 2003) published *Social Determinants of Health: The Solid Facts*, outlining a series of social factors that contribute to ill health. These included stress, social exclusion, work, unemployment, social support, addiction, food, and transportation. More recently, Marmot (2017, p. 690) placed particular emphasis on the need for a proper policy response and clarified that in order to reduce inequalities in health, broader social inequalities should be addressed, which basically reflect the models above about the causes of inequalities in health. He suggested the following: 'give every child the best start in life; education and lifelong learning; [improved] employment and working conditions; everybody should have the minimum income necessary for a healthy life; healthy and sustainable places to live and work'.

George: Nurse Kelly, are you sure about all this information?

Annette: As sure as I can be. Academics in the social sciences have been studying these dimensions for years and their findings are taught in medical and nursing schools. Believe it or not, there is scientific evidence that supports these theories.

George: I am completely depressed now.

Annette: Why? I thought that you would find this information useful.

George: Useful for whom exactly? You've basically said that I became sick and was hospitalised because I am poor. My father was poor, I did not complete my higher education, I smoke, and I drink. I feel as though I am being punished on account of things that I cannot control or that I enjoy doing.

Annette: You should not feel this way. Actually, you should take advantage of this new information and take the necessary actions recommended in order to protect yourself from developing chronic illness.

George: And it is not only this, it is also COVID-19. I am vaccinated and I have never been in close contact or had to isolate. With the number of new cases going up dramatically, I am terrified of becoming infected or a close contact and not being able to self-isolate so as to protect my family. We live in a small house. The protocol says that I have to self-isolate in my own house and avoid contact with the rest of the household. This is not possible. I am wondering what they were thinking when they came up with such a protocol. COVID-19 is affecting the whole planet, but it seems to me that the rich can better cope with the measures and protocols.

Annette: I know George. This is difficult for many people. You can check with the relevant department at the Ministry to see if they can accommodate you somewhere else.

George: I do not want to be away from my family. It would be worse.

DISCUSS

1. How could this sociological information assist George in improving his health?
2. What new social issues has George brought up?

GLOBAL HEALTH AND STRUCTURAL COMPETENCE

George's reference to COVID-19 pertains to the concept of global health. Global health relates to issues of determinants of health but at a global level. There are many definitions of global health in the literature, although there is not a consensus. In their systematic literature review, Salm et al. (2021) found 34 definitions of global health. A popular definition is from Koplan et al. (2009) who explained that

> global health is an area of study, research and practice that places a priority on improving health and achieving equity in health for all people worldwide. Global health emphasises transnational health issues, determinants and solutions; involves many disciplines within and beyond the health sciences and promotes interdisciplinary collaboration and is a synthesis of population-based prevention with individual-level clinical care.

In general, definitions of global health focus on health issues which concern all countries and responses should be global in order to provide solutions and ensure equity in all nations of the world.

Reflecting on the broad definition of the term, Harris and White (2019) conducted a literature review of the sociology of global health in order to identify key areas of concentration and research directions. They concluded that the key topics were relations and power, inequalities, gender, race, ethnicity and nationality, environment, culture, social movements, and organisations. An important question is how the world responds to global health problems or threats. Global response efforts have been informed by national, regional, or international organisations such as the World Health Organisation (WHO), Centers for Disease Control and Prevention (cdc.gov), European Medicines Agency (EMA), European Commission – Public Health, and so forth. These organisations can review and approve new medications and therapies as well as public health strategies for medical conditions which affect all people in the world or in specific geographical areas. Some examples include HIV/AIDS and Ebola. A more recent example is COVID-19. COVID-19 was initially identified in China in November 2019 and ever since it has affected the whole planet, forcing the WHO to declare it a pandemic in March 2020. Although there was no coordinated response to the COVID-19 pandemic, there were, initially, striking similarities across countries largely informed by recommendations by the WHO. Specifically, mass testing, isolation, social or physical distancing, lockdowns, use of masks, vaccination, etc., were among the measures that were observed in many countries around the world (Constantinou, 2021a). Another example of the global response to COVID-19 was the construction of a specific discourse which mainly presented COVID-19 as an enemy, focused on deaths and hospitalisations, punished those who violated the measures, emphasised the effectiveness of vaccines, and downplayed information pertinent to mild illness or asymptomatic patients and to problems of vaccines, etc. (Constantinou, 2022; 2021a; 2021b). Despite similarities in the responses to COVID-19 across countries, the global response did not seem to reflect global health coordination with agreed transnational objectives and outcomes. The global response failed in many terms, including measures which did not consider social inequalities and cultural understandings of the pandemic and vaccination, equal distribution of vaccines in all countries, addressing people's concerns, responding effectively to the psychosocial problems, or other health conditions resulting either from the pandemic itself or from the measures (Rollston and Galea, 2020).

Dealing with inequalities locally and globally is a complex and multidimensional issue, requiring policy response and individual actions (Marmot, 2020; 2017). Healthcare professionals could contribute to reducing inequalities by acquiring knowledge and skills in structural competence. Metzil and Hansen (2014) presented their proposal for moving from cultural competency to structural competency. They have defined structural competency as healthcare professionals' capacity to identify and respond to health and illness that are influenced by social, political, and economic structures. Social structures refer to 'the way a society is organised in hierarchies through institutions, policies, economic systems, and cultural or normative belief systems such as race, socioeconomic status, gender, and sexuality' (Bourgois et al., 2017, p. 300). Neff et al. (2017) considered structural competence essential for ensuring equality in healthcare, reducing health disparities, and addressing the issues of structural violence and structural vulnerability. Structural violence occurs when people are caused to be vulnerable by the social structures or arrangements they find themselves immersed into. Structural vulnerability is the risk for people to experience harm, resulting from structural violence.

Ensuring structural competence, Neff et al. (2017) carried on explaining that there are five skills that healthcare professionals should develop. These are: (1) recognise influences of structures on health, (2) recognise influences of structures on the clinical encounter, (3) respond to structures in the clinic, (4) respond to structures beyond the clinic, and (5) structural humility (collaboration with relevant stakeholder in order to respond to structural vulnerability effectively). Neff et al. outlined practical ways for clinicians to tackle inequalities, such as recognising the hierarchies and power relations involved in medical consultations, learn how to use existing services (e.g., interpreters), learn how to work effectively with behaviour and social services, create synergies with community representatives and community-based organisations to help patients from different cultural backgrounds, educate policymakers on patients' structural vulnerability, advocate for patients, etc. Neff et al. evaluated a structural competency programme by training 12 residents of the family residency programme in California. They found that the training helped them in practising medicine and working with diversity more effectively. Interestingly, being competent in identifying the structural influences on health was very overwhelming for them and they asked for further training so that they could be better equipped in terms of responding to these influences successfully.

REFERENCES

Action on smoking and health. *Health in Equalities and Smoking*; 2019. Available at: ASH-Briefing_Health-Inequalities.pdf.

Araki S, Murata K. Social life factors affecting the mortality of total Japanese population. *Soc Sci Med*. 1986; 23(11): 1163–9.

Bartley M, Blane D. Inequality and social class. In: Scambler G, editor. *Sociology as Applied to Medicine*, pp. 115–132. 6th ed. London: Saunders Elsevier; 2008.

Bartley M, Blane D, Smith CD. Introduction: Beyond the Black report. In: Bartley M, Blane D, Smith CD, editors. *The Sociology of Health Inequalities*, pp. 1–18. Oxford: Blackwell; 1998.

Blaxter M. *Health*. 2nd ed. Cambridge: Polity Press; 2010.

Bourgois P, Holmes SM, Sue K, Quesada J. Structural vulnerability: Operationalizing the concept to address health disparities in clinical care. *Acad Med*. 2017; 92(3): 299–307.

Bury M. *Health and Illness in a Changing Society*. New York: Routledge; 1997.

Case A, Deaton A. Rising morbidity and mortality in midlife among white non-Hispanic Americans in the 21st century. *Proc Natl Acad Sci USA*. 2015; 112(49): 15078–83.

Constantinou CS. 'Symbolic power' in COVID-19 field and language. *Hum Rev*. 2022; 11(1). https://doi.org/10.37467/gkarevhuman.v11.3080.

Constantinou, CS. Responses to COVID-19 as a form of 'biopower'. *Int Rev Sociol*. 2021a; 32(1): 29–39.

Constantinou CS. "People have to comply with the measures": Covid-19 in "Risk Society". *J Appl Soc Sci*. 2021b; 15(1): 3–11.

Donkin AJ. Social gradient. In: Cockerham WC, Dingwall R, Quah SR, editors. *The Wiley Blackwell Encyclopedia of Health, Illness, Behavior, and Society*. pp. 2172-2178. Chichester: John Wiley & Sons Ltd; 2014.

Elstad JI. The psycho-social perspective on social inequalities in health. *Sociol Health Illn*. 1998; 20(5): 598–618.

Enroth L, Fors S. Trends in the social class inequalities in disability and self-rated health: Repeated cross-sectional surveys from Finland and

Sweden 2001–2018. *Int J Public Health*. 2021; 66: 645513. doi: 10.3389/ijph.2021.645513.

Feinstein JS. The relationship between socioeconomic status and health: A review of the literature. *Milbank Q*. 1993; 71(2): 279–322.

Feldman JJ, Makuc DM, Kleinman JC, Cornoni-Huntley J. National trends in educational differentials in mortality. *Am J Epidemiol*. 1989; 129(5): 919–33.

Harris J, White A. The sociology of global health: A literature review. *Sociol Dev*. 2019; 5(1): 9–30.

Hu X, Wang T, Huang D, Wang Y, Li Q. Impact of social class on health: The mediating role of health self-management. *PLOS ONE*. 2021; 16(7): e0254692.

Kitagawa EM, Hauser PM. *Differential Mortality in the United States: A Study in Socioeconomic Epidemiology*. Cambridge, MA: Harvard University Press; 1973.

Koplan JP, Bond TC, Merson MH, et al. Towards a common definition of global health. *Lancet*. 2009; 373(9679): 1993–5.

Kunst AE, Looman C, Mackenbach J. Socio-economic mortality differences in the Netherlands in 1950–1984: A regional study of cause-specific mortality. *Soc Sci Med*. 1990; 31(2): 141–52.

Layte R, Whelan CT. Explaining social class inequalities in smoking: The role of education, self-efficacy, and deprivation. *Eur Sociol Rev*. 2009; 25(4): 399–410.

Loizos P, Constantinou C. Hearts, as well as minds: Wellbeing and illness among Greek Cypriot refugees. *J Refug Stud*. 2007; 20(1): 86–107.

Marmot M. The health gap: Doctors and the social determinants of health. *Scand J Public Health*. 2017; 45(7): 686–93.

Marmot M. Social determinants of health inequalities. *Lancet*. 2005; 365(9464): 1099–104.

Marmot M, Allen J, Boyce T, Goldblatt P, Morrison J. *Health Equity in England: The Marmot Review 10 Years On*. London: Institute of Health Equity; 2020. Available at: Health Equity in England_The Marmot Review 10 Years On_full report.pdf.

Marmot MG, McDowall ME. Mortality decline and widening social inequalities. *Lancet*. 1986; 2(8501): 274–6.

Metzl JM, Hansen H. Structural competency: Theorizing a new medical engagement with stigma and inequality. *Soc Sci Med*. 2014; 103: 126–33.

Neff J, Knight KR, Satterwhite S, Nelson N, Matthews J, Holmes SM. Teaching structure: A qualitative evaluation of a structural competency training for resident physicians. *J Gen Intern Med*. 2017; 32(4): 430.

Rogers A, Pilgrim D. *A Sociology of Mental Health and Illness*. 4th ed. Glasgow: Open University Press; 2010.

Rollston R, Galea S. The coronavirus does discriminate: How social conditions are shaping the COVID-19 pandemic. 2020. November 30, 2020. Available at: http://info.primarycare.hms.harvard.edu/blog/socialconditions-shape-covid.

Russell A. *The Social Basis of Medicine*. Singapore: Wiley-Blackwell; 2009.

Salm M, Ali M, Minihane M, Conrad P. Defining global health: Findings from a systematic review and thematic analysis of the literature. *BMJ Glob Health*. 2021; 6(6): e005292.

Silver M. An econometric analysis of spatial variations in mortality rates by race and sex. In: Fuchs VR, editor. *Essays in the Economics of Health and Medical Care*, pp. 161–209. New York: Columbia University Press; 1972.

Taylor S, Field D. *Sociology of Health and Health Care*. 4th ed. Singapore: Blackwell Publishing; 2007.

Townsend P, Davidson N. *Inequalities in Health: The Black Report and the Health Divide*. London: Penguin Books; 1990.

Van de Mheen HD, Stronks K, Mackenbach JP. A lifecourse perspective on socio-economic inequalities in health: The influence of childhood socio-economic conditions and selection processes. *Sociol Health Illn*. 1998; 20(5): 754–77.

Whitehead M. *The Health Divide*. London: Penguin Books; 1990.

Wilkinson R, Marmot M, editors. *Social Determinants of Health: The Solid Facts*. 2nd ed. Copenhagen: World Health Organization; 2003.

CHAPTER 7

Gender and health

....

ABSTRACT

Mr Graham Mayers is 60 years old. He and his wife visit their doctor for a routine check-up. The results show that he has elevated cholesterol levels and high blood pressure; however, his wife does not. He 'complains' to the nurse about the difference between men and women and begins a conversation by stating that the fact that women live longer and are healthier than men is simply not fair. The nurse, Fiona Peterson, does not agree with his views and presents some sociological theories that explain the existing distinctions that relate to gender and health. This chapter aims to help healthcare students and practitioners to gain a deeper understanding of the differences between men and women in health and illness, and work more effectively with gender identity.

LEARNING OBJECTIVES

- Describe the differences between men and women as these relate to mortality and life expectancy.
- Identify the difference between men and women as this relates to morbidity.
- Explain the reasons for the existing differences in life expectancy, mortality, and morbidity between men and women.

DOI: 10.1201/9781003256687-8

- Describe how masculinity and femininity may contribute to the ill health of men and women, respectively.

Note: Think about or discuss the questions that are in the boxes before you continue reading through the chapter.

SCENARIO

Mr Graham Mayers and his wife visit a local GP clinic for a routine check-up. Although his wife goes in for regular check-ups every six months, Graham rarely agrees to visit the doctor for a check-up. Finally, his wife convinces him to go to the GP clinic. While at the clinic, Nurse Fiona Peterson calls Graham into the examination room.

Fiona: Hello, Mr Mayers! Are you here for a routine check-up or have you been referred by your GP?
Graham [sarcastically]: I have been referred by my GP.
Fiona: Who is your GP?
Graham: My wife!
Fiona [laughs]: I see! Your wife persuaded you to come in for a check-up today.
Graham: Yes.
Fiona: Well, it really is for your own good that you are here today.
Graham: I was always wondering why women live longer than men and why they never get sick.
Fiona: I am not sure whether this is accurate, Graham. First let me take a small blood sample and measure your blood pressure and then we can have a little chat about the issues you have raised.

DISCUSS

1. What does Graham mean by stating that women live longer than men?
2. What does Graham mean by stating that women never get sick?
3. If both statements are indeed true, why is that the case?
4. What further information would you need from the relevant literature in order to answer these questions?

FURTHER DEVELOPMENTS

Graham returns the next day to discuss the results of his check-up.

Fiona: Graham, your blood pressure is 145 over 100. This is considered high. Is there anything that is currently making you stressed? Of course, your medical results will be reviewed by your GP.

Graham: I am not sure.

Fiona: From your blood work results, I see that your cholesterol is high as well. It is 300. Are you taking any medication for high blood pressure or high cholesterol?

Graham: No.

Fiona: OK, Graham, I would like you to tell me more about any past medical conditions you've had, as well as your family and social history.

Graham: I am not sure what you mean by all this but go ahead and ask me what you need to know.

Fiona: Have you suffered from any health conditions in the past?

Graham: Except for the occasional seasonal cold, no. Actually, I had surgery a long time ago to remove a benign tumour from one of my testicles. I don't have any chronic conditions, though.

Fiona: Do any of your close relatives suffer from any chronic illnesses that you know of?

Graham: Well, my brother has diabetes, but I believe that he is healthier than me since he isn't married.

Fiona: Type 1 or type 2 diabetes?

Graham: I do not know what the difference is; he got it when he was 30 years old.

Fiona: OK. Do you smoke, Graham? Or drink excessively?

Graham: I do both.

Fiona: How many cigarettes do you smoke per day?

Graham: About 15.

Fiona: And how many units of alcohol do you drink?

Graham: I drink three to five small glasses per day.

Fiona: Do you take any recreational drugs?

Graham: No, I don't.

Fiona: OK, Graham. Thank you for this information.

Graham: I know why you asked me about drinking and smoking. Both habits are 'medically fashionable' and if a doctor is not sure about the cause of a disease, then they immediately blame the existence of the condition on smoking and alcohol.

Fiona: No, that's not the case. There is scientific evidence that indicates the relationship of both smoking and drinking to ill health.

Graham: I am not sure if you have addressed my comment that women live longer, and they never get sick.

Fiona: What you are saying about the comparison between men and women is not entirely accurate. In fact, while research evidence shows that women indeed tend to outlive men, they are more likely to report being ill.

Graham: Why is this the case?

Fiona: That's a good question. Let me tell you some useful information that we learned from the social sciences we were taught at nursing school.

DISCUSS

1. What does Fiona mean by saying that women indeed live longer but are more likely to report ill health?
2. What are the most important reasons for these differences?

HEALTH DIFFERENCES BETWEEN MEN AND WOMEN

Women live longer than men. This is a fact in many, but not all, Western countries. Scambler (2008) explained that this was not always the case in Europe. In the 16th and 17th centuries, men had longer life expectancies, but this began to change in the early 19th century, and by the early 20th century, women were outliving men. The reason why women died younger in the 16th and 17th centuries had to do with mortality rates at childbirth and the fact that women were more likely than men to die from the deadly diseases affecting people at that time, such as tuberculosis, typhus, and typhoid fever. Modern industrialisation and urban living, interestingly, benefited women more than men and, therefore, a change was observed from the early 20th century onwards (Scambler, 2008).

Scambler (2008) illustrated that in the UK, in 1901, men were expected to live until the age of 45 years, while women were likely to live until the age of 49. This four-year difference remained stable over the years, in spite of the increase in life expectancy for both men and women. More specifically, in the UK in 2005, men's life expectancy was 77 years and women's was 81 years. The largest variation between men and women in terms of life expectancy was witnessed in 1969 and was 6.3 years. Since the 1980s, this difference has been decreasing; however, women continue to live longer than men.

A critical question to be asked is whether men and women die from similar causes. If yes, do these causes occur to the same extent in both genders? According to the *Statistical Bulletin* (ONS, 2011), heart disease, cancer, and respiratory diseases are the three most common causes of death for both men and women. However, men are more likely than women to die from these causes. In other words, these conditions are more likely to develop in men than in women. Taylor and Field (2007) outlined the findings of studies that compared women and men with regards to lung cancer, heart disease, and skin cancer. They noted that lung cancer was more prevalent among men in 1974; however, this gap became increasingly narrower by 2002. This was attributed to the smoking rates among men and women and the fact that, by then, more women smoked than ever before and, moreover, they were smoking almost as much as men were.

The same studies identified that heart disease was the main cause of death for both men and women, but men were more likely than women to die from it. However, this difference could be attributed to gender patterns in smoking, as well as age, as men smoke more than women do when they get older (Taylor and Field, 2007). A recent report by the Office of National Statistics in the UK (2020) showed that ischaemic heart disease was the leading cause of death among men, while the leading cause of death for women was dementia and Alzheimer's disease. In support, Gao et al. (2019) showed that men were more likely than women to have a heart disease, however, the interpretation of data should be approached carefully. Women develop heart disease later in life and when they do develop acute cardiovascular incidents, they are more likely to have a poor prognosis. Interestingly, more women are likely to suffer from skin cancer (though the gap between men and women is narrowing), though more men die from the disease. Research has shown that men tend not to take the risk of sun exposure seriously, and that women are more likely than men to take measures to protect themselves from the sun's ultraviolet radiation (e.g., the use of sun creams).

Given all this, the question that arises is why do these differences in life expectancy and mortality exist between men and women, and does biology alone account for these differences? There are many social factors that play a role in creating differences in life expectancy and mortality (Courtenay, 2000; Nettleton, 2006; Scambler, 2008; Russell, 2009). *First*, the type of job performed by an individual has had an impact. That is, historically, men have been engaged in more dangerous professions, such as underground mining, fishing, working in the construction industry, and so forth (Bird et al., 2012). *Second*, men are more likely than women to be engaged in dangerous activities or hobbies. For example, car racing, extreme sports, driving while under the influence of alcohol, and so on. *Third*, men are more likely than women to be involved in criminal activities and, thus, are at greater risk of being attacked or harmed by other people. *Fourth*, men that suffer from a health condition or illness tend to delay seeking help and, as a result, the disease is allowed to spread and cause further damage or harm. *Fifth*, women are more likely than men to follow healthier lifestyles. These are the main social factors that have had an impact on male and female life expectancies. The reason why men engage in such behaviours is addressed later in the chapter and relates to the issue of masculinity and femininity. Moreover, smoking and drinking have been associated with ill health and patterns of use differ between men and women. The 2020 report on smoking in the UK by the Office of the National Statistics showed that men still smoked more than women, although the gap was not great (15.9% vs 12.5%). Zambon (2021) also explained that men consumed more strong alcoholic drinks than women in the UK and they are also more frequent drinkers. Interestingly, significantly more men than women exceeded the drinking limit per week. More specifically, in age groups 45–64 and 65+, 37% of men compared to 19% of women, and 33% of men compared to 14% of women, respectively, exceed drinking limits. In addition, more alcohol-specific deaths were observed among men than among women (Zambon, 2021).

Fiona: So you see, Graham, based on these research findings, you possess some of the characteristics and behaviours that are understood to contribute to the lower life expectancy of men. You are a heavy smoker and drinker and, therefore, you have a greater risk of developing a cardiovascular disease or lung disorder, compared to your wife who has never smoked. Also, you do not undergo regular check-ups, which can assist in identifying an illness or health condition in its early stages. Instead, your wife has to persuade you to come in for a check-up.

On this note, could men be more likely than women to fall sick? The popular research finding is that women are more likely than men to be sick; however, this is based on self-reported data. Basically, this means that women are more likely than men to report having poor health.

Furthermore, they are more likely to seek medical help and consultation and are more likely to report symptoms (Bayram et al., 2015; Case and Paxson, 2005; Scambler, 2008).

Graham: Yes, but this does not mean that women tend to get sick more
often than men.
Fiona: You are correct.

Research evidence is largely based on self-reported data and concludes that, taking into consideration all health conditions, women are more likely than men to suffer from ill health, though not necessarily from life-threatening conditions (Taylor and Field, 2007; Scambler, 2008). However, the literature shows that women are more likely than men to report their illness. More specifically, the 2004 General Household Survey (cited in Taylor and Field, 2007) showed that women reported more limiting, long-standing illness and health-related restricted activity, but the difference between the two genders was not statistically significant. Interestingly, women over 65 years old were more likely than men to report health-related restricted activities. Taylor and Field attributed this difference to the increased incidence of arthritis and rheumatism in women. Along similar lines, Macintyre et al. (1999) studied men and women's patterns of reporting their health conditions and, through the use of open-ended questions, found that men were more likely to give more elaborate accounts of their health. The authors did not put forward this finding in order to argue that men reported illnesses more frequently but rather that men were just as likely as women to report their health conditions.

There are many explanations for the difference in reported morbidity between men and women. Taylor and Field (2007) explained that, out of the general data, two main approaches emerged as reasons for these observed differences. *First*, women are indeed more likely than men to suffer from illnesses. Bartley (cited in Taylor and Field, 2007) compared men and women, aged 20–60 years old, and found that women were more likely than men to have minor psychological conditions, though both men and women demonstrated similar patterns during the assessment of their general health. Men suffered from serious chronic conditions (such as heart disease) more often (Riska, 2012), and while women seemed to have higher rates of morbidity, they were statistically higher than those of men. In support, women might be more likely to have less serious conditions (such as arthritis), which might contribute to a poorer self-health assessment (Molarius and Janson, 2002). *Second*, the difference between men and women resulted from the women's tendency to report illnesses more frequently, rather than suffering from higher rates of morbidity as compared to men. Spiers et al. (2003) maintained that women might be more eager to share any symptoms they may recognise. This also meant that men were less likely to pay attention to symptoms, report them, and consequently, seek medical help (Idler, 2003). The above has been supported by a recent study which indicated that women made more visits to doctors than men, but this was largely driven by frequent gynaecological issues women would like addressed (Byram et al., 2015).

FURTHER DEVELOPMENTS

Fiona outlined the findings above and went on to explain to Graham that masculinity and femininity are also important factors which account for the difference in health between the two genders.

Fiona: Graham, you are right to point out that women tend to consult their doctors more easily or readily and that this does not necessarily mean that they get sick more often than men. This is because women tend to recognise symptoms quicker than men and, as a result, they look for help during the early stages of a disease. Women, however, are more likely to suffer from psychological conditions, while men are more likely to suffer from serious chronic conditions, such as heart disease and lung cancer. This fact contributes to the increased mortality rates among men.

Graham: I see!

Fiona: The fact that men tend to suffer more often from chronic diseases does not account for the difference in life expectancy and mortality rates. As I already explained, there are many social factors that impact this, and these have to do with the differences in lifestyle among men and women as well as the higher risk activities that men tend to engage in.

Graham: That makes sense.

Fiona: This is largely due to the masculine identity of men and the feminine identity of women. From a very young age, men and women are socialised to assume their respective identities, which appear to be responsible for a lot of the health-related behaviour practised by the two genders.

Graham: What exactly do you mean by saying that we are socialised with either a masculine or feminine identity? I do not understand. Men are men and women are women. Naturally, we are born different.

DISCUSS

1. What is masculinity and femininity?
2. How do they relate to ill health?

MASCULINITY, FEMININITY, AND ILL HEALTH

Fiona: I completely disagree with you! Certainly, there are biological differences between the two sexes but there are no biological reasons behind many of the roles that men and women undertake in society.

Graham: What do you mean exactly? Could you provide me with an example?

Fiona: Let me explain in more detail.

Masculinity and femininity are social identities, which are constructed by cultures in order to organise social environments, classify and control human behaviour and, thus, define men and women as acceptable social beings (Annandale and Hunt, 1990). Though masculinity and femininity vary across countries, nevertheless, they serve the same function. That is, to set a series of criteria in order to define, understand, and evaluate men and women. These identities are not fixed but instead they are processes that start before the actual event of childbirth. In modern Western societies, male and female identities come into play from the moment that the sex of the fetus is announced. Upon learning the sex of their baby, parents usually prepare for their future newborn by buying clothes and toys, decorating the nursery and so forth. All of these actions are not free of value; rather, they are contexts of identity on which culture begins inscribing its rules. For example, the colour blue is typically associated with baby boys and pink with girls. The nurseries of baby boys are decorated with cars or wild animals, whereas princesses and flowers will feature as decorative themes of nurseries designed for baby girls. Toys are gendered, too. Parents, relatives, and friends tend to purchase violent or aggressive toys, such as sport cars and soldiers for boys, while the toys girls play with, such as dolls and model kitchens, are designed to socialise girls with the values of taking care of a home and family. Such differentiation among genders occurs on many levels, including ways of dressing, styles of walking, expression of emotions and so on (Brody, 2000). In other words, gendered segregation is witnessed from very early on in life, so that human beings learn about, and embody, different social roles and behaviours, to the extent that they become second nature and evolve as an integral part of a person's self.

This gender role segregation continues into childhood, adolescence, and adulthood. Boys play different games compared to girls, which are typically more aggressive. Moreover, they are encouraged to pursue specific subjects in school, which have been termed 'hard subjects', such as science, physics, maths, and the like, whereas girls are encouraged to pursue 'soft courses', such as literature and history. There are cultures that have a predefined turning point from childhood into manhood, and a ritual is associated with this transition. Van Gennep (1960) has called this a 'rite of passage', in which a person is isolated from the community, undergoes a process of transition or an ordeal and, finally, is reincorporated into the community in a different, usually higher, social status. The main reason these rites of passage are tough is because some cultures view them as a way to separate the boy from the female world of his mother and therefore the ordeal has to be tough in order to give more importance to the separation from the female world, which is understood to be smooth and tender (Bowie, 2000). In some modern societies, the army functions as a rite of passage to manhood and group membership (Winslow, 1999).

Later in life, men are more likely than women to be the sole breadwinners, hold the top managerial positions in the labour market, and earn higher salaries than women. In general, men are socially viewed as being strong, calm, possessing material resources and self-control, as well as ultimate control of their family. Social expectations for women differ and have to do with taking on a caring and nurturing role and freely expressing their feelings. Although in modern, Western societies women are expected to work, it is more acceptable for women to be unemployed than it is for men.

Graham: OK, I understand the point that you are trying to make, and I agree with some of the observations you have made. However, even if you are absolutely correct, what does all this have to do with the health of men and women?

Fiona: Well, Graham, you may not realise it yet, but this information is directly linked to gender and health!

Connell (1995, pp. 77–9) argued that there were main masculinities, which related to different levels of power. The first one was 'hegemonic masculinity', which encompassed power in the workplace, physical strength, and heterosexuality. The next form of masculinity was 'complicit masculinity', which was close to hegemonic masculinity but did not have all of its benefits. The third type of masculinity, 'subordinated masculinity', included homosexuality, and worked as a context for devaluing men. Courtenay (2000) in his article, 'Constructions of Masculinity and Their Influence on Men's Well-Being: A Theory of Gender and Health', relied on Connell's hierarchy of masculinity to assert that men wished to achieve hegemonic masculinity, which was the ideal form in which to be socially accepted as a man. Health beliefs and behaviour turned out to be a manifestation of this pursuit. More specifically, Courtenay noticed that men were less likely to express and share their needs and inform others about their weakness and vulnerability. Instead, men were likely to consider asking for help as a feminine trait and, thus, would avoid doing so. In contrast, in an attempt to highlight their masculinity, men might refuse to take any sick leave, as work was considered a context in which they could construct and reaffirm their masculine identity. Similarly, men might insist that they do not need many hours of sleep in order to be strong, or that alcohol does not impact their driving abilities. Furthermore, men might avoid using sunscreen, thus placing themselves at a greater risk of developing skin cancer. Applying sunscreen would violate many of the masculine criteria, such as their perceived resistance to illness and their strong physique and would make them seem feminine. The onset of a disease might be devastating for men because it can disrupt their perceived power and possession of hegemonic masculinity. They might, for example, keep their medical condition under wraps and continue working long hours in order to prevent the disruption of their masculine identity.

To achieve hegemonic masculinity, men tend to be involved in risky or health-harming behaviours. To illustrate, men are more likely than women to smoke, abuse alcohol, and drive while intoxicated (see also Scambler, 2008). As a result, men are more vulnerable to diseases associated with smoking and alcohol abuse, such as lung cancer and liver disease, respectively. Smoking and alcohol consumption have been associated with masculinity as they are regarded as 'hard' pastimes and, thus, are regarded by many societies as male habits. Interestingly, the gap in smoking rates between men and women is narrowing, as women are increasingly adopting traditional male habits (Cockerham, 2007).

However, it is not solely smoking and alcohol that place men at a greater risk of developing chronic disease or of dying at a younger age than women. Men are more likely to be involved in dangerous activities, such as motorbike racing and climbing; they tend to drive more dangerously than women and, as a result, are more likely to be injured in car accidents (Barry and Yuill, 2016). All these activities have a common quality and cultural value, that of power and strength, which societies have traditionally viewed as masculine characteristics. Other behaviours that are associated with power include holding back or suppressing one's feelings and the need to feel as though one has total control of one's life. In failing to do so, a man may be regarded as vulnerable or weak and, as a result, may be considered as feminine.

Graham: I still do not quite understand what you are trying to say. Is it that men engage in such high-risk behaviours in order to reaffirm their masculine identity?

Fiona: Not exactly. Allow me to elaborate further.

Men do not engage in such behaviours because they want to prove that they are men. By performing these activities, men reaffirm their masculine identity; however, this is the aim of such activities, not the motive. Men are socialised from an early age to be strong and powerful. As they grow older, these values become second nature and, later in life, they pursue occupations and hobbies that support these values. Simply put, they choose these pastimes because they enjoy them (as these activities align with their cultural and cognitive map), and the function or outcome of performing these activities is to reaffirm their masculine identity. Courtenay (2000) went on to explain that men did not behave in certain ways merely because they wanted to achieve hegemonic masculinity, but also because they did not wish to be associated with the feminine identity. Expressing their feelings, showing their vulnerability, actively seeking help, avoiding risky behaviours, and so forth, would indicate that men were veering towards the feminine side.

Cameron and Bernardes (1998) presented qualitative data to further explain masculine behaviour in terms of dealing with health problems related to the prostate. Their data showed that men considered health to be the responsibility of women. As such, they avoided disclosing whether or not they had a problem with their prostate, they thought that health promotion was a female task and that suffering from a prostate problem threatened their masculine identity. Cameron and Bernardes presented specific examples to illustrate these points. *First*, they found that men did not talk about health as much as their wives did and they actually let their wives do the health-related talking. *Second*, men not only delayed seeking medical help but, in some cases, they may hide their health condition. The authors presented the example of a man with prostate disease who avoided disclosing his condition to his wife because he thought he could handle his problem on his own. *Third*, the reason why men were not involved in promoting their health was due to the perceptions that this act was purely feminine and did not fall under masculine activities and characteristics. *Fourth*, prostate problems were understood as a threat to the masculine identity as it disrupted men's lifestyles, impacting work, family life, and daily activities. Prostate problems also had an impact on sexual activity, which both younger and older patients considered to be a fundamental part of their masculine identity. A recent qualitative study by Noval et al. (2019) showed similar results and concluded that seeking help was influenced by perceived masculine values such as self-reliance, independence, and stoicism.

Updated research evidence presented in this chapter showed that various behaviours by men indicate masculinity as a possible underlying force (Zambon, 2021; Office of National Statistics, 2020; Barry and Yuill, 2016; Byram et al., 2015). These behaviours include smoking, drinking, avoiding seeking medical help, and dangerous and criminal activities. However, understanding the exact relationship between masculinity and ill health is lacking in the published literature (Ragonese and Barker, 2019; Etienne, 2019).

FURTHER DEVELOPMENTS

Fiona attempts to convince Graham that his smoking and drinking habits, while reaffirming his masculinity, negatively affect his health and that he should consider putting an end to them if he wants to live a healthier life.

Fiona: So, Graham, let me summarise. It is true that women outlive men, but this has been the case since the early 20th century – it was not true before then. The good news is that the gap between men's and women's life expectancies is increasingly narrowing. Heart disease and cancer are the main causes of death among both men and women, but heart disease and lung cancer are more prevalent among men. Women tend to report more often that their health is not good, and they report more chronic diseases. This does not necessarily mean that they are sicker but that they tend to report their illnesses more frequently. Moreover, they are more likely than men to recognise symptoms and are therefore more likely to seek help. Interestingly, they seem to suffer more from mental disorders.

Graham: Thank you, Fiona. Though I still don't agree with everything that sociology presents about the role of men and women in society,

I now understand the general picture that relates to health between the two genders.

Fiona: Well, Graham, since you cannot do anything about the biological differences between you and women in order to narrow down the gap in mortality and morbidity, you can certainly do something about the social differences.

Graham: What do you mean?

Fiona: For example, you could stop, or at least reduce, your smoking and drinking.

Graham: But I enjoy these activities and they help me relax and get away from my wife's nagging.

Fiona: Of course. You know now that you like smoking and drinking possibly because you have been socialised with the values that underline these habits. Consider whether you would still enjoy them, or even try them, if you were socialised with different values? Maybe not. I know it is not easy to change your habits and perceptions after so many years of being conditioned to think and behave in this way; however, we can discuss how we can help and support you to change these habits.

Graham: I must admit that your overview of how men and women are socialised demonstrates the impact of society on people's attitudes and behaviour. It is not easy to change, but I can try to reduce both my smoking and drinking gradually so that I can take the time to get used to the new lifestyle.

Fiona: This is a good way to go and certainly safer than doing nothing.

FURTHER DEVELOPMENTS

Fiona calls her colleagues for a meeting to discuss her encounter with Graham. She thinks that all patients, patients' relatives, and health professionals could be trained to recognise the underlying values of their masculine and feminine behaviour and how this behaviour could potentially influence their health and their health-related behaviour. Fiona's suggestions are well received and there are now plans to form a new department that focuses on health training and development at the GP clinic.

REFERENCES

Annandale E, Hunt K. Masculinity, femininity and sex: An exploration of their relative contribution to explaining gender differences in health. *Sociol Health Illn.* 1990; 12(1): 24–46.

Barry AM, Yuill C. *Understanding the Sociology of Health*. 4th ed. London: Sage; 2016.

Bayram C, Pollack A, Wong C, Britt H. Obstetric and gynaecological problems in Australian general practice. *Aust Fam Physician*. 2015; 44(7): 443–46.

Bird CE, Lang ME, Rieker PP. Changing gendered patterns on morbidity and mortality. In: Kuhlmann E, Annandale E, editors. *The Palgrave Handbook of Gender and Healthcare*, pp. 145–61. 2nd ed. London: Palgrave Macmillan; 2012.

Bowie F. *The Anthropology of Religion: An Introduction*. Oxford: Blackwell Publishing; 2000.

Brody LR. The socialization of gender differences in emotional expression: Display rules, infant temperament, and differentiation. In: Fischer AH, editor. *Gender and Emotion: Social Psychological Perspectives*, pp. 24–47. Cambridge: Cambridge University Press; 2000.

Cameron E, Bernardes J. Gender and disadvantage in health: Men's health for a change. *Sociol Health Illn*. 1998; 20(5): 673–93.

Case A, Paxson C. Sex differences in morbidity and mortality. *Demography* 2005; 42(2): 189–214.

Cockerham WC. *Social Causes of Health and Disease*. Cambridge: Polity Press; 2007.

Connell RW. *Masculinities*. 2nd ed. Berkeley, CA: University of California Press; 1995.

Courtenay WH. Constructions of masculinity and their influence on men's well-being: A theory of gender and health. *Soc Sci Med*. 2000; 50(10): 1385–401.

Etienne CF. Addressing masculinity and men's health to advance universal health and gender equality. *Revista Panamericana de Salud Pública*. 2019; 42: e196.

Gao Z, Chen Z, Sun A, Deng X. Gender differences in cardiovascular disease. *Medicine in Novel Technology and Devices* 2019; 4: 100025.

Idler EL. Discussion: Gender differences in self-rated health, in mortality, and in the relationship between the two. *Gerontologist*. 2003; 43(3): 372–75.

Macintyre S, Ford G, Hunt K. Do women over-report morbidity? Men's and women's responses to structured prompting on a standard question on long standing illness. *Soc Sci Med*. 1999; 48(1): 89–98.

Molarius A, Janson S. Self-rated health, chronic diseases, and symptoms among middle-aged and elderly men and women. *J Clin Epidemiol*. 2002; 55(4): 364–70.

Nettleton S. *The Sociology of Health and Illness*. 2nd ed. Cambridge: Polity Press; 2006.

Novak JR, Peak T, Gast J, Arnell M. Associations between masculine norms and health-care utilization in highly religious, heterosexual men. *Am J Men's Health*. 2019; 13(3), 1557988319856739.

Office of the National Statistics. *Adult Smoking Habits in the UK: 2019*; 2020. Available at: Adult smoking habits in the UK 2019(1).pdf.

Office of the National Statistics. *Leading Causes of Death, UK: 2011–2018*; 2020. Available at: Leading causes of death, UK 2001 to 2018.pdf.

Office of the National Statistics. *Statistical Bulletin: Deaths registered in England and Wales*; 2011. Available at: www.ons.gov.uk/ons/dcp171778_284566.pdf.

Ragonese C, Barker G. Understanding masculinities to improve men's health. *Lancet*. 2019; 394(10194): 198–9.

Riska E. Coronary heart disease: Gendered public health discourses. In: Kuhlmann E, Annandale E, editors. *The Palgrave Handbook of Gender and Healthcare*, pp. 178–91. 2nd ed. London: Palgrave Macmillan; 2012.

Russell A. *The Social Basis of Medicine*. Singapore: Wiley-Blackwell; 2009.

Scambler A. Women and health. In: Scambler G, editor. *Sociology as Applied to Medicine*, pp. 133–58. London: Saunders Elsevier; 2008.

Spiers N, Jagger C, Clarke M, Arthur A. Are gender differences in the relationship between self-rated health and mortality enduring? Results from three birth cohorts in Melton Mowbray, United Kingdom. *Gerontologist*. 2003; 43(3): 406–11.

Taylor S, Field D. *Sociology of Health and Health Care*. 4th ed. Singapore: Blackwell Publishing; 2007.

Van Gennep A. *The Rites of Passage*. London: Routledge & Kegan Paul; 1960.

Winslow D. Rite of passage and group bonding in the Canadian Airborne. *Armed Forces & Society* 1999; 25(3): 429–57.

Zambon NP. *Alcohol Statistics: England*; 2021. Available at: CBP-7626.pdf (parliament.uk).

CHAPTER 8

Ethnicity and health

ABSTRACT

Mr Anup Banerjee is a 52-year-old migrant who moved to England from Bangladesh 20 years ago. He is a poor man, who is married without any children. He arranged a meeting with a GP to undergo some medical tests due to some chest pain that he has been experiencing for a while. He talks to two nurses who think that migrants become sick due to genetics and lifestyle; however, he does not seem to endorse such explanations. Anup believes that he became ill because of the chronic stress he has been experiencing and due to the racism to which he has been exposed. This chapter aims to help healthcare students and practitioners to understand the concepts of race and ethnicity, their relationship with ill health, and to acquire more knowledge and skills in working more effectively with patients from diverse ethnic backgrounds.

LEARNING OBJECTIVES

- Describe the meaning of race and ethnicity.
- Outline the social conditions of migrants in their host country.
- Describe the differences in health conditions between migrants and native people.

DOI: 10.1201/9781003256687-9

- Describe any variations in health conditions across ethnic groups.
- Explain the social basis of migrants' health conditions.

Note: Think about or discuss the questions that appear in boxes before you continue reading through the chapter.

SCENARIO

Mr Anup Banerjee arranged a meeting with a GP to undergo some medical tests due to chest pains that he has been experiencing for the last few months. He had arranged an appointment for Monday at four o'clock in the afternoon. By quarter to five, he had been waiting for nearly an hour and no one had approached him to inform him when the doctor would be able to see him. He is angry and begins to think that he is being discriminated against due to his race. He wonders to himself, 'Would I have to wait for so long if I was a White man named Steve?' He sees two nurses at the end of the corridor looking at him and talking to each other in a low voice.

Nurse Penny Williams: Do you know what he is here for?

Nurse Alisa Morgan: No, he is a foreigner, maybe an Indian. You know these people tend to have specific diseases due to their genetics. They may die younger or have chronic conditions that result from genetics and cultural habits, such as diet. Even their eating habits are influenced by their genes.

Penny: Yes, I know. Did the doctor tell you when he would be able to see the patient?

Alisa: No, he has to wait a while because there are many patients waiting to see the doctor. Let's talk to him for a while.

Alisa and Penny approach Anup.

Penny: Hello, how are you today? What is your name?

Anup: I am Anup Banerjee. I am OK, but I have been waiting for almost one hour to see the doctor.

Alisa: Yes, the doctor has many patients to see today, and I am afraid that you will have to wait a little while longer.

Penny: Anup, do you come from India?

Anup [tensely as he found the question irrelevant]: Do I look like an Indian? I come from Bangladesh. And for your information, I feel, think, and act like a Bangladeshi. When is the doctor going to see me? It seems to me that the coloured patients are the ones waiting to see the doctor, while the White people are being called in.

Alisa: Don't worry, Anup. Since you made an appointment, your turn will come soon.

DISCUSS

1. Why did Alisa and Penny assume that Anup came from India? What sociological terms could be used to explain their assumption?
2. What does Anup's statement about 'feeling, thinking, and acting like a Bangladeshi' refer to?

RACE AND ETHNICITY

Alisa and Penny immediately assumed that Anup was from India possibly based on his outward appearance and they attributed his possible health condition to his genetic make-up. Essentially, Alisa and Penny have made a presumption about Anup's health condition on the basis of race, which refers to the categorisation of people on account of shared biological characteristics, such as skin colour and general physical appearance (Kelly and Nazroo, 2008). Laypeople and, very often, health professionals share a common approach to race, assuming that people from different countries have distinct genes, which are responsible for specific diseases that are not so common in their home countries. The concept of race goes hand in hand with widely held stereotypes about people from other places. Stereotypes are widely held beliefs about shared characteristics and behaviour of people that belong to the same group (Greenwald et al., 2002). In other words, stereotypes about the British, for example, may state that the British are reserved and distant. People then use these stereotypes to assume that all British people possess these characteristics and behaviour. Stereotypes are used in all cultures and are very powerful as they serve certain functions. *First*, they simplify people's complex and busy world. *Second*, they facilitate people's understanding of their surroundings and people's predictions for the future. Stereotypes, thereafter, reinforce assumptions about race and the pre-existing concept of race activates and reinforces stereotypes. Alisa and Penny utilised the concept of stereotypes to form certain assumptions about Anup's health. They initially assumed that Anup did not differ from other people from India and, subsequently, they tried to explain his possible health condition using his race. Though they touch on culture by bringing up Anup's eating habits, they actually attribute everyone's dietary habits to genetics, thus reinforcing their assumptions about race.

Categorisation is also used institutionally for statistical and research purposes, as well as for policymaking, as is the case with the UK National Health Service (NHS). This provides a way to monitor access and improve treatment. For example, the NHS uses the following categorisation: White, Mixed, Asian, Asian British/Scottish (Indian, Pakistani, Bangladeshi, other Asian), Black or Black British/Scottish (Black Caribbean, Black African, Black other), Chinese, Other (Kelly and Nazroo, 2008, p. 162). This categorisation differs across countries, though it does not necessarily relate to how people understand themselves and it does not account for mixed ethnic backgrounds. Such categorisation, though still prominent in the NHS, might be problematic for research purposes and, as a result, for policymaking because it is does not reflect reality and may result in wrong policy decisions (Kelly and Nazroo, 2008).

Interestingly, though Anup would possibly tick 'Bangladeshi' if completing an NHS form, without much thought, he found Alisa and Penny's bold assumption about his background odd and he felt the need to clarify his ethnicity and culture. These two terms are not one and the same. There are many definitions of culture and in this case Tylor's definition is presented which, referring to 'culture, or civilisation, taken in its broad, ethnographic sense, is that complex whole which includes knowledge, belief, art, morals, law, custom, and any other capabilities and habits acquired by man as a member of society' (Tylor, 1958, p. 1). In other words, culture refers to any products (or actions) that result from human action, from clothing to language, and from the production of objects to customs and rituals. Ethnicity relies on cultural characteristics people share, which form the basis for constructing their own identity and the image in the eyes of others who are either members of the group or outsiders (Cohen, 1985). Anup's response and reaction to Alisa and Penny are manifestations of both ethnicity and culture.

To emphasise his ethnicity, Anup stresses his place of origin, a fundamental context in which people share values, beliefs, and behaviour, and develop their sense of belonging. To link ethnicity with cultural aspects, Anup highlights that his feelings, thoughts, and actions are similar to those of other Bangladeshi people. Basically, Anup uses the cultural characteristics he believes he shares with other people to support his ethnic background. However, Anup does not only pay attention to what he shares with other Bangladeshis, but also to what he does not have in common with people who do not belong to his ethnic group. His question, 'Do I look like an Indian?' is reminiscent of Cohen's (1985) approach to community construction. Cohen argued that people constructed their communities through various means. *First*, people developed a sense of belonging through shared values, beliefs, behaviours, and customs. *Second*, people's sense of belonging was reinforced when they could identify differences in the values, beliefs, behaviours, and customs of other groups. Thereafter, creating a sense of belonging was a comparative process. *Third*, people's sense of belonging was solidified through the construction of an external enemy, which strengthened collective awareness of their group's characteristics and increased their integration. Anup activated the first two means outlined by Cohen. That is, he emphasised what he has in common with other Bangladeshis and he indirectly compared Indians with Bangladeshis in order to further clarify the groups' differences and, thus, strengthen the uniqueness of people from Bangladesh.

FURTHER DEVELOPMENTS

Alisa: What brings you here today, Anup?

Anup: I have been having chest pains for the past few months and I thought it would be a good idea to consult with a doctor.

Penny: It could be nothing serious. However, it could be a more serious condition with your heart. Migrants usually have such problems.

Anup: Why do you think that migrants are more likely to have heart problems?

Penny: Well, genetics can play a role, as well as certain habits, such as diet.

Anup: I find that hard to believe! For starters, the British eat more fattening food than we do.

Alisa: That might be the case, Anup. However, genes can play a very powerful role in determining whether an individual might be at risk of developing certain diseases.

DISCUSS

1. What are the main health conditions affecting migrants in Western countries?
2. Do migrants' health conditions differ to those of local people? If yes, why is this the case?
3. Are there any differences across ethnic groups?

At that moment, Natalie McLaren, a third-year medical student, passes by and happens to overhear part of the conversation. She decides to interrupt the conversation. Given that the sociology material she was taught at medical school is still fresh in her mind, she feels confident enough to correct both Alisa and Penny, who either have been wrongly informed or rely heavily on their personal opinions which seem to be informed by cultural stereotypes.

Natalie: I am sorry to intrude, but I think it is useful to understand the social conditions under which migrants live, and gauge their general health profile, before we can understand if, and why, their health differs from that of White British people.

Initially, Alisa and Penny look at Natalie with a doubtful expression on their faces. Nevertheless, they indicate that they are interested to hear what she has to say and, so, they encourage her to continue.

Natalie: I am sure that you will find what I am about to tell you to be very enlightening.

MIGRANTS' SOCIAL CONDITIONS AND HEALTH PROFILES IN WESTERN COUNTRIES

Alisa and Penny made two assumptions, which have been documented by Gupta et al. (1995). They attributed the high rates of coronary disease found among South Asians to genetics and diet. Gupta et al. argued that to reduce the rates of coronary disease, South Asians living in Britain could be educated so as to be better informed of healthier eating habits and about the importance of physical exercise so that they could reduce related risk factors. The question that arises here is how far are diet and lifestyle associated with the health of migrants in Western countries? Are there any other social factors that play a role in the health profiles of migrants? To answer these questions sufficiently, we need to explore the social conditions affecting migrants in their host country, as well as their general health profiles.

Vast numbers of individuals migrated to Western countries, such as the UK, after World War II due to the increased need for labour. As a result, people from the Caribbean, South Asia, and Ireland moved to the UK in the 1950s and 1960s; during the following decades, individuals immigrated to the UK from Bangladesh, Pakistan, and India. Individuals from Ghana, Turkey, Sri Lanka, and Somalia moved to the UK just before the 21st century. The 2001 Census revealed that these migrants made up 7.9% of the UK population (Kelly and Nazroo, 2008). What social conditions have these migrants been subjected to?

The Office of National Statistics indicated that the majority of migrants resided in urban areas. Migrants tended to live with their families; family size varied across ethnic groups, with Bangladeshi families having on average 4.5 members, while families from the Caribbean represented the smallest family unit with only 2.3 members (Kelly and Nazroo, 2008). Interestingly, a similar trend was observed in household income, based on data from the Office of National Statistics. That is, while 21% of White families were categorised as living with low income, this percentage was higher among migrants: 30% of Indian, 31% of Caribbean, 49% of Black other, and 68% of Bangladeshi and Pakistani immigrants fell into the low-income category. Kelly and Nazroo (2008) explained that the ethnic groups who were financially closer to the White population were the Indian and the Chinese populations. In general, migrants in the UK tended to have big families and poor financial resources, with Bangladeshi migrants being in the worst position.

However, what is the general health profile of migrants in the UK? Kelly and Nazroo (2008) described and summarised the statistics published by the Office of National Statistics in the UK from 1991 to 1993. Caribbean men had low mortality rates due to coronary diseases and were more likely to die from a stroke than from any other disease. Interestingly, people from West and South Africa displayed a similar trend in terms of coronary disease and stroke but, in general, had high mortality rates. People from Bangladesh were more likely than other ethnic groups to die of coronary disease; people from India presented high rates of death from a stroke; while migrants from Ireland indicated high mortality rates due to strokes, coronary problems, respiratory diseases, and lung cancer. Interestingly, Becares (2015) discussed variation in the health profile of ethnic groups. There were groups that fared better than the White British such as Chinese, Black African, and Indian. However, Black Caribbean, Arab, Bangladeshi, Pakistani, and White Gypsy, or Irish Travellers, especially women, had worse health. The three ethnic groups which had the worst rates in limiting long-term illness among people from the age group 16–64 were Bangladeshi, Pakistani, and White Gypsy or Irish Travellers for both genders. Updated reports published in 2021 confirm these findings (Raleigh and Holmes, 2021). A similar variation was identified in the United States, where Hispanic, Black, American Indian, and Alaska Natives reported the worst health (Artiga et al., 2016). Khanijahani et al.'s (2021) systematic review showed that ethnic minority groups were affected the most during the COVID-19 pandemic as they were more likely to become infected, be hospitalised, and die.

The information presented above seems to neither support genetics nor lifestyle in explaining migrants' health. Though genetics and lifestyle do have an impact on people's health condition, they cannot adequately explain the variations across ethnic groups. Social scientists need to consider other social factors that could potentially cause this difference.

DISCUSS

1. Why does the data above fail to support genetics and lifestyle as possible causes of ill health experienced by migrants?
2. What other social reasons might influence the ill health of migrants?

FURTHER DEVELOPMENTS

Alisa: Yes. However, this information does not completely rule out genetics, correct?

Natalie: No, though it provides you with a context for understanding any other social reasons that might be responsible.

Alisa: Anup, we think it is genetics and lifestyle. What do you think are the reasons for your ill health?

Anup: No, it is not genetics. If it were genetics, then all Bangladeshis would have the same health problems and to the same extent. This is not the case. I know people my age who have never been sick and others that have already passed away from cancer, heart attacks, and strokes. I think the two reasons that I am sick has to do with constant stress and racism. We live in a racist country, ladies!

Penny: What do you mean? Everyone living in the UK has equal access to health services. According to your patient file, I noticed that you live in a community that consists of more British residents than migrants.

Anup: Yes, but I have been waiting here for more than one hour now, and I still haven't been able to see the doctor. It seems to me that your British fellow citizens do not have this problem. I have been a victim of racism many times: at the supermarket, on the bus … even in parks when I take time out to walk around and relax.

Penny: What is it exactly that makes you feel so stressed, Anup?

Anup: The need to survive; to have the necessary financial means. Racist behaviour and social exclusion also make me feel uncertain about the future. I try to socialise with other Bangladeshis so as to feel a greater sense of belonging; however, it does not always work as I spend most of my time with British people.

Alisa: Anup, the doctor is ready to see you now.

Anup: Finally! He must have finished seeing all the White patients! [*Anup smiles and treats his comment as a joke.*]

Dr Philip Peterson: Good afternoon, Mr Banerjee. How are you today?

Anup: Hello, Doctor. I am OK, but I have been having chest pain and sometimes I also experience breathlessness, and this has been going on for some time now.

Dr Philip: Alright, let me examine you first and then you will need to have a series of medical tests.

>   *Dr Philip examines Anup.*

Dr Philip: I can hear some arrhythmias. You do not need to worry about this for now as it may not be anything serious. Let's administer the medical test first and schedule another appointment one week from now when we have the results.

>   *Anup returns after a week and, once again, has to wait for one hour and 15 minutes before he is able to see the doctor. By this time, he has become frustrated and stressed, but he needs to visit the doctor in order to find out what is affecting his health.*

Dr Philip: Welcome back, Anup. How are you today? Do you feel better?

Anup: Yes, Doctor, thank you! Do you have my test results?

Dr Philip: The results show that you have a coronary problem. Basically, two central valves have closed to the extent that medical intervention is required.

Anup: What exactly do you mean?

Dr Philip: Well, to start with, you will need to take some medication, which I will prescribe for you now. At the same time, you need to make some changes to your lifestyle, as well as your diet to minimise your risk of suffering from a heart attack.

Anup: Do you have any suggestions as to what I could do to reduce the stress and racism that I experience as a result of living in this country?

Dr Philip: Anup, it seems to me that you might benefit from talking to a professional. You need to find ways in which to cope with that fact that you live in a foreign country. If you like, I could refer you to our psychologist who might be able to assist you with any psychosocial concerns that you may have.

Anup: I am not sure if this would help as I believe that society needs to change, not me!

DISCUSS

1. What does Anup mean when he says, 'society needs to change'?
2. How can modern society influence people's health?
3. What does Anup mean by stating that he may have a heart problem on account of his chronic stress?
4. Why does Anup think that racism is the main cause of his ill health? What is racism and what forms could it take in health settings?

Natalie, who observed the medical consultation, was eager to talk to Dr Peterson about the medical sociology knowledge she recently acquired and that she believes could shed some light on Anup's case and support his claim that modern society was to blame for the ill health experiences of migrants. Dr Peterson, who had not had the opportunity to pursue any sociology courses at the medical school he graduated from, was curious to find out more.

Dr Philip: Natalie, you are here to learn but, at the same time, you could teach us one or two things! If you have any information that could help us better understand our patients, and thus support us in our task of helping them improve their health, then please feel free to share this information with us.

MIGRANTS' SOCIOECONOMIC STATUS AND HEALTH

The relevant literature does not seem to regard genetics or lifestyle as the prominent factors that could explain the difference in health between migrants and native people. Social scientists, therefore, have paid more attention to the general socioeconomic status of migrants and examined the relationship between socioeconomic inequalities and migrants' health. Given the observation that migrants are not a unified group but, rather, that health varies across ethnic groups, Kelly and Nazroo (2008) examined statistical data within ethnic groups and found that, among all the main ethnic groups residing in the UK (Caribbean, Indian, Pakistani, Bangladeshi, Chinese and, White non-British), those with a better socio-economic status were healthier; while those who indicated the lowest income were significantly more likely to report poor health. Thereafter, ethnicity per se did not seem to be the foremost reason accounting for this difference. In other words, if ethnic background was the main factor, greater homogeneity within groups would be observed.

Cooper (2002) studied the relationship between reported health, gender, and ethnic background by analysing data collected through the Health Survey for England (HSE) spanning the period from 1993 to 1996. The author managed to obtain 43,500 responses from people aged between 20 and 60 years old. Cooper found that about 20% of Pakistani and Bangladeshi men were unemployed, while the percentage of Pakistani and Bangladeshi women who had never worked was almost 60%. This meant that these two ethnic groups were more likely to be disadvantaged in terms of household income and resources. Not surprisingly, these groups reported poor health. However, socioeconomic status was not the main factor affecting health among all ethnic groups, as explained below.

White (2009) analysed the case of the Australian Aborigines in order to illustrate that the socioeconomic factor, per se, did not account for the health profile of an ethnic group. Aborigines and Torres Strait Islanders in Australia demonstrated striking differences in health compared to other ethnic groups. More specifically, Aborigines and non-Aboriginal Australians had similar life expectancies only when taking into consideration the life expectancy of non-Aboriginal Australians 100 years ago. This meant that the main improvements in living conditions, which largely accounted for the increase in life expectancy, had not yet been experienced by the Aborigines. Compared to the general population, life expectancy between 1998 and 2000 was 20 years lower among men and 21 years lower among women. Furthermore, the mortality rates of infants in the Aboriginal population were significantly higher than those of non-Aboriginal Australian infants. Interestingly, Aboriginal children were more likely than non-Aboriginal Australian children to be hospitalised and, additionally, they were more likely to die during hospitalisation. The socioeconomic status of the Aborigines was much lower than that of the general population, though White stressed that this alone did not sufficiently account for such great differences. Therefore, White outlined a number of possible reasons for these differences. *First*, Aborigines were more exposed to risks that result from pollution, environmental hazards, and injuries at work. *Second*, Aborigines had a low social status within Australian society, which might have resulted in chronic stress. *Third*, Aborigines were more likely to die from serious chronic diseases, such as heart disease, diabetes, and tuberculosis. The reason for this had to do with the fact that these conditions went undetected and untreated. Besides the socioeconomic status of the Aborigines, there might be other factors that contributed to their health problems. To elaborate, lack of financial resources, education, health awareness, and exposure to racism might be contributing factors to the generally disadvantageous health status among Aborigines.

Drawing from the studies presented in the previous sections about the health profile of the Bangladeshi, Pakistani, and White Gypsy or Irish Travellers population in the UK, a report by the British government showed that these three ethnic groups had the highest percentages for routine occupations or had never worked, indicating their poor socioeconomic status (Socioeconomic Status, 2020). Therefore, it seems that low socioeconomic background should be considered for explaining the health profile of ethnic minority groups. However, more recent research has highlighted the complexity of the issue as data shows that it is not socioeconomic status per se but an array of factors, which need to be understood in relation to race and ethnicity (Williams, Priest, and Anderson, 2016). For example, the difference in heart disease between Blacks and Whites is smaller than the educational gap between the two groups. Along similar lines, Assari, Caldwell, and Bazargan (2019) found that improving parents' educational attainment had a positive impact on outcome for youth; yet this was true only for the Hispanic group but not for the non-Hispanic group. Williams, Priest, and Anderson (2016) stressed the need to look at other aspects such as life-course, racism, psychosocial stress, problematic socioeconomic indicators which may not capture adequately the differences in financial hardships. Assari, Caldwell, and Bazargan (2019, p. 10) emphasised that 'it is race/ethnicity and class, not race/ethnicity or class, that affect health disparities'.

One of the social experiences that might result in chronic stress is racism. Racism was used as a possible explanation by Farmer and Ferraro (2005), who studied the relationship between reported health and socioeconomic status and ethnicity in the United States. They found that Black American adults were more likely to suffer from serious diseases and less likely to report good health as compared to Caucasian adults. Interestingly, high socioeconomic status was not found to offer the same benefit. That is, though Black adults from a higher socioeconomic status were more likely than those from a lower socioeconomic status to report their health as good, they were more likely to report bad health compared to their Caucasian counterparts. Farmer and Ferraro attributed this to the racist experiences that Black adults experienced in American society and to the possibility that Black adults embodied the disadvantages they experienced on account of racism and, in turn, transformed these disadvantages into poor self-reports about their health. Ethnic groups might experience racism at many levels and in many instances within everyday life, and in this case, within the medical treatment they are subjected to. The health implications of racism are discussed in the following section.

Dr Philip: So, Natalie, in order to make sure that I understood you clearly, allow me to summarise. Poverty and socioeconomic status are contributing factors affecting the health of migrants; however, they are not the only ones. Social conditions and experiences (such as the presence of social support networks) could play a role, correct?
Natalie: Exactly, racism also seems to have a strong impact on the well-being of migrants.
Dr Philip: In what way?

RACISM, INSTITUTIONALISED RACISM, AND MIGRANTS' HEALTH

Kelly and Nazroo (2008) considered racism as a social factor with important implications on the health of ethnic groups. In the United States, inequalities in access and treatment to healthcare have been observed due to differences in healthcare insurance benefits (see also Nazroo and Williams, 2005). In the United Kingdom, no serious inequalities should be expected in terms of access to healthcare due to the openness of the NHS. However, Kelly and Nazroo (2008) observed that inequalities in the UK were found in the quality of care and treatment. More specifically, ethnic minority groups were more likely to negatively evaluate the care they received, reporting issues relating to waiting time and communication problems with health professionals due to language barriers. These experiences pertain to the term 'institutionalised racism', which refers to any form of informal discrimination on the basis of race and ethnicity at an institutional level (Taylor and Field, 2007, pp. 86, 89). Institutional racism could occur in organisations, such as schools, hospitals, governmental departments, and so forth, and could be direct or indirect. Direct institutional racism refers to an overt discriminating policy that an organisation may adopt in order to exclude foreign people from gaining access to the available services. For example, excluding Black people from accessing specific healthcare settings. Indirect institutional racism refers to a covert form of discrimination, which may be a remnant of direct racism or a form of racism that acquires a symbolic form. That is, delaying the medical appointments of foreign people, in spite of the absence of a formal institutional policy, indirectly promotes racist behaviour. Another example of indirect institutional racism is employing teachers who have not received any training in multicultural education techniques in areas where poor people or migrants reside.

Though robust research in the relationship between racism and health in the UK is scarce, Karlsen and Nazroo's (2002) study aimed to shed light on the relationship between racism and health. Karlsen and Nazroo relied on the Fourth National Survey of Ethnic Minorities (FNS) in order to explore the implication of racism on health. The FNS utilised a representative sample of 5,196 people from the Caribbean and Asia, and 2,867 White people. All participants completed a face-to-face structured interview and were classified into ethnic groups based on their family origins. The study revealed that experienced racism had a significant impact on how ethnic minority groups reported their health. That is, those who were victims of racism were 55% to 125% more likely to describe their health as poor. Karlsen and Nazroo explained that their study was supported by other past studies which showed a relationship between racism and stress, heart disease, as well as ill physical and mental health.

Integrating the research findings, Kelly and Nazroo (2018) came up with a diagram which depicted the role of a series of social factors that may influence an individual's health. At the centre of the diagram is the individual who is affected by genetics, age, and gender. Beyond the individual, participation in social groups, such as religion, family, friends, and the community, played a significant role. Other significant factors were education, housing, employment, healthcare treatment, healthcare prevention, and institutional racism. Four forces finally had an impact on people's health. These were social structure, cultural competence, racism, and culture. Cultural competence referred to 'the capacity to provide effective healthcare taking into consideration people's cultural beliefs, behaviours, and needs' (Papadopoulos, 2003, p. 5, cited in Kelly and Nazroo, 2008, p. 197). Basically, cultural competence represented a cultural way to deal with racism and institutional racism.

The question that arises is where can Anup be found within this model? Though we do not know about Anup's genetic profile and how this might have an impact on his health, male gender and middle age are two individual characteristics that could influence Anup's lifestyle and health behaviour. However, Anup has been affected by other forces as well. He does not seem to have many friends around and he lives in an area where the majority of residents are native British. This means that Anup experienced limited participation in migrant communities and is exposed to many incidents of racism. He also falls within a lower socio-economic status and is uneducated. The former factor places Anup at the risk of developing serious chronic diseases and dying at a younger age, while the latter makes him less likely to be informed about health issues. Finally, Anup is experiencing institutionalised racism at the GP clinic he visited.

Another critical question here is what can be done to improve Anup's health? A few ways pertain to structural competence (covered in Chapter 6) and these are: *First*, he would benefit from improving his awareness of the impact of cultural beliefs and health behaviour (Kelly and Nazroo, 2018). On this note, informative or educational campaigns about healthier lifestyles would be beneficial. *Second*, he could be trained so as to find a better job and move upwards in the socioeconomic strata. *Third*, in order to deal with racism, Anup could relocate to an area inhabited by Bangladeshi migrants. This would reduce stress and boost feelings of belonging, as well as self-esteem and value. In such communities, people feel integrated into the group; they participate in activities and lead more meaningful lives (Nazroo and Williams, 2005). *Fourth*, institutional racism could be tackled by governments and relevant laws, while institutions should be under constant surveillance and subject to quality assurance control by external bodies, which would address issues related to racism. Furthermore, institutional leaders and managers should be made aware of institutional racism, because lack of awareness or ignorance may be the reason behind a lack of change or improvement. Paradies et al.'s (2015) systematic review and meta-analysis found a clear link between racism and poor mental and physical health. Interestingly, there was variation in the sense that the impact of racism on mental health was greater for Asian Americans and Latino Americans than for African Americans.

Dr Philip: Thank you, Natalie. This is well-presented information that is very helpful. It would be impossible for either of us to completely change society and make the world a fair place for everyone. However, we do have a responsibility to make sure that health professionals are aware of the research results you have presented. In this way, they would be able to improve their communication skills with patients and explore how institutional procedures could be adapted or developed so as to improve the health condition of migrants, as well as the quality of medical treatment offered to them.

Do you think that Anup has been a victim of institutional racism by our clinic?

Natalie: Yes, I think he has. He arranged a visit with you two weeks ago. He arrived at the clinic and had to wait for over an hour to see you. In the meantime, he observed many White British patients being called in for check-up and treatment. I am not saying that the clinic has a formal policy on appointments and waiting times for migrants and native people but perhaps, subconsciously, the secretaries who handle the appointments consider the health conditions of migrants to be less important. Whatever the case, it would be a useful exercise to examine our existing procedures and current practices so as to identify ways in which we could improve on the medical treatment of patients who are migrants.

FURTHER DEVELOPMENTS

Having informed her GP supervisor, Dr Philip Peterson, that the hospital appears to support equal opportunity on paper, by allowing equal access to all people including migrants, Natalie noted that she had observed certain inadvertent actions that could be considered racist. On this note, Natalie suggests that the hospital should review its procedures in order to deal with covert institutionalised racism and secure equal treatment. Furthermore, Natalie informs her supervisors that some nurses have false perceptions and general stereotypes about the health of migrants and, thus, they sometimes communicate with patients in an inappropriate way. Dr Peterson is quickly convinced that staff require training and begins to organise a workshop that will include participation by social scientists and health policy consultants. Such a development would ensure that the hospital staff and procedures are culturally and structurally competent (see Chapter 1 for cultural competence, and Chapter 6 for structural competence).

REFERENCES

Artiga S, Foutz J, Cornachione E, Garfield R. *Key Facts on Health and Health Care by Race and Ethnicity*. Kaiser Family Foundation; 2016. Available at: https://www.kff.org/racial-equity-and-health-policy/report/key-facts-on-health-and-health-care-by-race-and-ethnicity/.

Assari S, Caldwell CH, Bazargan M. Association between parental educational attainment and youth outcomes and role of race/ethnicity. *JAMA Network Open*. 2019; 2(11): e1916018.

Becares L. Which ethnic groups have the poorest health. *Ethnic Identity and Inequalities in Britain: The Dynamics of Diversity*; 2015; 123.

Cohen AP. *The Symbolic Construction of Community.* London: Ellis Horwood Ltd and Tavistock Publications Ltd; 1985.

Cooper H. Investigating socio-economic explanations for gender and ethnic inequalities in health. *Soc Sci Med.* 2002; 54(5): 693–706.

Farmer MM, Ferraro KF. Are racial disparities in health conditional on socioeconomic status? *Soc Sci Med.* 2005; 60(1): 191–204.

Greenwald AG, Banaji MR, Rudman LA, Farnham SD, Nosek BA, Mellott DS. A unified theory of implicit attitudes, stereotypes, self-esteem, and self-concept. *Psychol Rev.* 2002; 109(1): 3–25.

Gupta S, De Belder A, Hughes LO. Avoiding premature coronary deaths in Asians in Britain. *BMJ.* 1995; 311(7012): 1035–6.

Karlsen S, Nazroo JY. Relation between racial discrimination, social class, and health among ethnic minority groups. *Am J Public Health.* 2002; 92(4): 624–31.

Kelly M, Nazroo J. Ethnicity and health. In: Scambler G. *Sociology as Applied to Medicine*, pp. 159–75. London: Saunders Elsevier; 2008.

Kelly M, Nazroo J. Ethnicity and health. In: Scambler G, editor. *Sociology as Applied to Medicine*, pp. 179–202. 7th ed. London: Saunders Elsevier; 2018.

Khanijahani A, Iezadi S, Gholipour K, Azami-Aghdash S, Naghibi D. A systematic review of racial/ethnic and socioeconomic disparities in COVID-19. *Int J Equity Health.* 2021; 20(1), 1–30.

Nazroo JY, Williams DR. The social determination of ethnic/racial inequalities in health. In: Marmot M, Wilkinson RG, editors. *Social Determinants of Health*, pp. 238–266. 2nd ed. Oxford: Oxford University Press; 2005.

Papadopoulos R. The Papadopoulos, Tilki and Taylor model for the development of cultural competence in nursing. *JHSEI.* 2003; 4(1): 5–7.

Paradies Y, Ben J, Denson N, Elias A, Priest N, Pieterse A, ... Gee G. Racism as a determinant of health: A systematic review and meta-analysis. *PLOS ONE.* 2015; 10(9): e0138511.

Raleigh V, Holmes J. The health of people from ethnic minority groups in England. *The King's Fund*; 2021. Available at: The health of people from ethnic minority groups in England | The King's Fund (kingsfund.org.uk).

Socioeconomic Status. *Gov UK, Ethnicity, Facts, Figures*; 2020. Available at: Socioeconomic status — GOV.UK Ethnicity facts and figures (ethnicity-facts-figures.service.gov.uk).

Taylor S, Field D. *Sociology of Health and Health Care.* 4th ed. Singapore: Blackwell Publishing; 2007.

Tylor E. *Primitive Culture.* New York: Harper & Row Publishers; 1958.

White K. *An Introduction to the Sociology of Health and Illness.* 2nd ed. London: Sage; 2009.

Williams DR, Priest N, Anderson NB. Understanding associations among race, socioeconomic status, and health: Patterns and prospects. *Health Psychol.* 2016; 35(4): 407.

CHAPTER 9

Ageing society and older people

....

ABSTRACT

Mr David Gordon is 80 years old and suffers from bowel cancer and a cardio-vascular condition. He visits the doctor for routine check-ups and to monitor his conditions. Although David does well, his cancer relapses with metastasis, causing the condition to have a poor prognosis. His wife would like to take care of him, but she does not want the doctor to inform David about the prognosis. This chapter aims to help healthcare students and practitioners to understand the social aspects of ageing, better appreciate the impact of medical conditions on older people, informal care, death and dying, and the importance of cultural competence in building a good relationship with the patient and their relatives.

LEARNING OBJECTIVES

- Explain the terms demographic transition and rectangularisation of the life curve.
- Describe the term ageing society.
- Outline the approaches to the socialisation of ageing.
- Explain the terms life-course and structural dependency.
- Define informal care and outline the needs of individuals who provide informal care.

DOI: 10.1201/9781003256687-10

- Explain the relationship between social class, ethnicity, and informal care.
- Describe social death, changes in people's perceptions of death, awareness contexts, and good death.

Note: Think about or discuss the questions that appear in boxes before you continue reading through the chapter.

SCENARIO

Mr David Gordon is 80 years old and suffers from bowel cancer and has had a cardiovascular condition for 18 years. He visits Dr Michael Shepard in order to undergo routine check-ups and to monitor his condition. He has been suffering from bowel cancer for three years now. David is a talkative type of person and starts asking the doctor why people nowadays have so many diseases. He continues saying that he remembers when he was a child and his mother told him that people did not have many diseases in the past. Dr Shepard explains that people live longer now than ever before, but David says that diseases are everywhere.

DISCUSS

1. What does David mean when he says that 'nowadays people have so many diseases'?
2. Why does the doctor say that people live longer now than ever before?
3. What further information from the literature do you need in order to answer these questions?

DEMOGRAPHIC TRANSITION

David believes that, in the past, people did not suffer from so many diseases and, as a result, they were more content. Naturally, David does not rely on scientific evidence to formulate such a view and, instead, he romanticises the past as compared to the present, which is full of risks and where people suffer from chronic conditions. While it is documented that nowadays there are more chronic conditions than ever before, it is also recognised that these chronic conditions are largely the result of ageing and the fact that people live longer than ever before (Taylor and Field, 2007).

David is 80 years old. At the time he was born in Britain in 1933, only about 30% of individuals reached the age of 80 (Higgs, 2008). Over time, the percentage of people who lived until the age of 80 increased to about 70%. So, if David was born earlier, in the 1920s for example, his chances of reaching 80 years old would be smaller. In the UK, life expectancy in 1841 was 41 years for men and 43 years for women; while, in 2005, life expectancy was 77 and 81 for men and women, respectively. This time trend has been presented through the 'rectangularization of the life curve in England and Wales' (Higgs, 2008, p. 177), which showed that, in 2011, the curve would almost form a rectangular shape.

A rectangular shape means that living until the age of 70 is almost certainly due to decreased infant mortality and an increase in the number of years lived. Due to this rectangularisation of the life curve, interesting demographic changes have been observed. According to Xu et al. (2010), the percentage of people who are 65 years and older has dramatically increased, while the percentage of people under the age of 16 has decreased. This is a result of people living longer nowadays and, thus, increasingly, people are reaching the age of 65 or older. More specifically, in 1900 in the United States, there were 3.1 million people over the age of 65, but 100 years later this number had reached 35 million, and it is expected to double by 2030 (Harris, 2007). Simultaneously, birth rates in Western countries have dropped significantly, as couples are choosing to have fewer children.

In the intervening years between 1900 and 2030, the percentage of people who were 65 years and older increased at a constant rate; this is a phenomenon known in the United States as 'the greying of America' (Harris, 2007, p. 26). Harris explained that there were three main indicators of an ageing society. *First*, the percentage of older people increased. *Second*, the ratio of older-to-younger people was growing. *Third*, the median age, which separated the age of the population into two segments, increased. A way to represent this graphically is through the construction of a 'population pyramid' (Harris, 2007, pp. 27–8), which compares the proportions of age populations. However, there was another reason for the phenomenon of the rising percentage of older persons: a demographic baby boom. A baby boom period refers to a historical period during which the number of newborns is disproportionately higher than that witnessed during other historical periods. A baby boom occurred in the United States after the World War II largely due to the economic growth that followed and, as a result, 76 million children were born between 1946 and 1964. This generation has been called the 'boomer generation' (Harris, 2007, p. 29) and people born during this period are expected to turn 65 during the 2010s and 2020s.

This has led to a phenomenon that has been called 'the ageing society' (Taylor and Field, 2007, p. 114). Interestingly, this demographic transition has brought about new challenges in modern society, which relate to the management and treatment of health conditions among the elderly, as well as the social conditions that older people face.

HEALTH AND ILLNESS IN OLDER AGE

David has conditions that typically affect many people over the age of 65. The Office of National Statistics in the UK published data regarding how people of different ages understood their health (Higgs, 2008). The distinction was between chronic illness and restrictive chronic illness. The data showed that both chronic illness and restrictive chronic illness increased as age advanced, while the most commonly reported chronic health conditions experienced in older age were arthritis, back pains, heart disease, and mental illnesses. Interestingly, it was observed that, though people nowadays live longer than ever before, this does not necessarily mean that they live a healthy life until they pass away at an older age. More specifically, Higgs went on to explain that life expectancy among men in 2002 was 76 years; however, the number of years for healthy life expectancy was almost 10 years lower (67.2 years old). In other words, people were expected to live without any disabilities for 60 years but were likely to spend 15 years living with a disability. In 1981, a similar trend was witnessed, although the number of years people were expected to live with a disability was 12.8. This means that over time people may live longer but they will spend more years being sick. David was 62 years old when he was diagnosed with a cardiovascular condition and three years ago developed bowel cancer. Therefore, he has spent the past 18 years living with health conditions that have impeded his lifestyle. This represents a long period of time, which has allowed him to develop a thorough understanding of the restrictions resulting from his condition, as well as to formulate an opinion about the psychosocial anguish experienced after retirement (see Chapter 2 for more about embodiment).

In 1995, in his article 'Ageing, Meaning and the Allocation of Resources', Moody published four scenarios about the future of old age. He postulated the 'prolongation of morbidity', in which people would live longer but would not necessarily be healthy. Conversely, 'the compression of morbidity' was a state whereby many people enjoyed a healthy life until the end of their lives. Moody also wrote about 'prolongevity: life extension' and 'recovery of the life-world'. In the former situation, people would live even longer, while in the latter, individuals would need to acknowledge the restrictions brought about through ageing and take necessary actions for the benefit of both the older and younger generations. David falls mainly in Moody's prolongation of the morbidity scenario, in the sense that he is 80 years old but these last two decades have not been accompanied by good health given his cardiovascular disease. To this end, David does not represent a suitable example of Moody's compression of morbidity as his morbidity has not been condensed.

SOCIAL CONDITIONS IN OLDER AGE

Older people tend to live in nuclear families or alone, while many of them reside below the poverty line. Higgs (2008), referring primarily to the UK, explained that women outlived their husbands and, given the observation that women often chose not to marry again, older people tended to live alone. However, the majority of them had grown-up children who resided in areas nearby and, thus, maintained frequent contact with them. Therefore, though older people tended to live alone, they had important social contacts – their children and grandchildren. By the same token, older people constructed social networks with friends and neighbours. Interestingly, when in need, older people received informal care from these social networks. In spite of the social networks that older people could draw from, they nevertheless found themselves at risk of poverty related to retirement and the subsequent reduction in income (Age UK, 2016).

In the EU, the dominant definition of poverty is that of relative poverty, which refers to determining whether someone lives in poverty in relation to other people in the same country. In other words, relative poverty compares citizens living in the same country to determine who is poor and who is not. The threshold has been set at 60% below the median income in a country (Marx and Van den Bosch, 2000). According to results among EU countries (Antczak and Zaidi, 2016), the average percentage of older people who are at risk of poverty varies across countries with the EU being 17.8%. Bulgaria, Latvia, Estonia, and Romania have the highest percentages of older people living at risk of poverty, while Denmark, France, the Netherlands, and Luxembourg have the lowest. Echoing the data above, Burholt et al. (2020) discussed a number of risks older people may be faced with which may potentially cause them to be more vulnerable to exclusion from social relations. These are personal attributes, physical risk, retirement, socioeconomic status, exclusion from material resources, and migration.

Interestingly, caution should be taken when trying to present the social circumstances facing the elderly in modern societies. Usually, social scientists pay attention to majorities and general trends in the population to highlight the social disadvantages of older people. However, Harris (2007) explained that the majority of people who have the greatest power, who enjoy the highest social status and are the richest people in modern societies, are older people. Therefore, old age does not always represent a context associated with disadvantage and helplessness; rather it can provide a framework for exercising power that derives from the possession of financial means and political strength.

FURTHER DEVELOPMENTS

Dr Michael: David, could you please let me know how you cope with the conditions in your life.

David: I am alright for the time being. I am glad I am clean from cancer and my Alzheimer's is mild. However, I am sad I am not doing what I used to before retirement.

Dr Michael: Could you please tell me more?

David: I was very active before retirement; I was a teacher, working long hours. I felt useful and strong. Following my retirement, I fell into a state of mild depression since it seemed that society expected me to withdraw from the labour force simply because I had reached the age set for retirement. In reality, I felt as though, by retiring, I had lost access to one of the main structures that gave meaning to my life – my job. I felt terrible when I had to leave my teaching position. Soon after, I felt even more useless when the government took over my life!

Dr Michael: What do you mean by 'the government took over your life'?

David: Well, ever since my retirement, I must rely on the government for my pension, access to healthcare, and other services. All this makes me feel useless; I am completely dependent on the government.

Dr Michael: I see. What do you do to pass your time on a day-to-day basis?

David: For the time being I am focused on changing my lifestyle; I plan on altering everything from my diet to my wardrobe! I want nothing associated with old age in my life. I want to change my appearance and lifestyle. I want to wear jeans and exercise. Since my cardiovascular condition is stable and my cancer has not come back, I am OK; I do not feel old. What does 'old' mean anyway?

DISCUSS

1. Why does David feel that retirement is a negative experience?
2. What does his reference to the role of the government refer to?
3. Why does David want to alter his lifestyle at the age of 80?

SOCIALISATION AND AGEING

David has highlighted one of the most important roles he had in his life, that of teacher, through which he acted and socialised further. However, what is the importance of a social role and why was being a teacher so important to David? Social roles are an integral part of socialisation, which is a very dynamic and powerful process (Giddens, 2006). It is basically a process through which people learn the rules of behaviour in a given culture. In other words, socialisation is the process of learning about a culture, which refers to customs, ways of life, dress code, facial expressions, body language, civilisation, values, rules of behaviour, and so forth. A key component of socialisation is the roles people are expected to perform throughout their lives in order to achieve their personal and cultural goals. For example, being an employee is a social role, which means that an employee is expected to act in certain ways in accordance with the rules and expectations of the organisation in which they are employed. An example of a cultural goal would be to be a well-paid employee who would be able to live independently or support a family (cultural values), while a personal goal would be to make money and be well respected as a successful employee within the workplace and the wider community.

Thereafter, social roles are contexts for action and construction of our social identity – what defines us as social beings. Through long-term immersion of people in their social roles, they end up defining and presenting themselves according to their roles (that is, I am a sociologist, I am a father, and so forth). David, as a teacher, represents an example of a person who had thrown himself into the role of teaching for so many years that, in turn, he lived for this role. Moreover, he was regarded as a successful teacher by his peers and students and, as a result, teaching became more than just a job. It became a framework through which

David defined himself as a social individual. It was a characteristic of his total self. Losing this identity framework upon retirement was problematic for David, as he had to find other frameworks for his actions and self-affirmation.

Old age is a period when people are made to abandon or change some of their roles or undertake new ones. These roles include those of employee, manager, parent, husband, wife, and so forth. Harris (2007, pp. 82–7) outlined a few approaches to reconsidering roles during old age. *First,* 'role loss' may occur on account of retirement, widowhood, and the deterioration of health. *Second,* the 'disengagement theory' explained that there has been a gradual withdrawal of older people from their social roles and both society and older people were preparing to dissociate from one another. Such disengagement might be functional in the sense that older people retreated and provided the younger generations the space, power, and opportunity to manage society. In other words, society needs younger people in order to maintain its order. *Third,* according to the 'continuity theory', older people continued their previous ways of life and they depended on their past experiences in order to continue their socialisation. *Fourth,* the 'activity theory' presented the elderly as active agents; not in the sense that they continued their social roles, but in the sense that they were actively trying to find new roles to compensate for the loss of the previous roles held. In this case, society distanced itself from the individual (not vice versa) and the individual tried to deal with this separation by finding new social contexts for socialisation. *Fifth,* 'role ambiguity' might be experienced after retirement, widowhood, or diagnosis with a chronic disease when the person was confused and there were no clear boundaries of the role they were supposed and expected to perform. *Sixth,* 'role discontinuity' referred to a state in which people stopped preparing to enter into a new role. Before retirement, people very often took actions to prepare the ground for taking on a new role. For example, an individual might improve their professional skills to secure a promotion or a new job, meaning that they continued assuming new roles. However, during retirement, older people might stop taking any steps to aid them in taking on new roles.

Interestingly, David's experience could be applied to more than one of these approaches, such as role loss, role discontinuity, activity theory, and continuity theory. That is, David lost his role as a teacher upon retirement, and he withdrew from his role since he was too depressed and frustrated to continue. However, he now wants to take on new roles to change his appearance and feel young again. In other words, he wants to be active and resume a past role. Such role taking and continuity could work well for David, both psychosocially and biologically. The implications of socialisation and role taking have been documented (Hall-Lande, 2007); they lead to a healthier psychosocial state and function as protective factors against isolation, depression, and general biological deterioration. When older people are psychosocially active, they keep their body busy and their general health is likely to improve (Ageuk, 2016; Ahlskog et al., 2011; Fried et al., 2004).

Interestingly, David's retirement has raised another issue. He complains that the state does everything for him now; implying that he depends solely on the state for his survival. David's experience has been represented by the term 'structured dependency' (Townsend, 1981, p. 23). This term drew attention to the role of social policy and any changes in policy that place older people under the auspices of the state. This means that the state determines the age of retirement and the onset of pension. In other words, older people are structurally made to leave their former work activities and, consequently, must depend on the state in order to survive. As explained above, one of the social groups that are likely to be below the poverty line is that of people older than the age of 65. This was the case since older people were made to abandon the labour force and were forced to become dependent on a low pension by which they were expected to manage their financial needs. However, limited financial means may have left many older people socially inactive, or at least not as active as they would like to be. Such a structural approach to old age has led to a form of discrimination against the elderly in the sense that emphasis and value have been placed on younger generations.

CULTURES OF AGEING

David has gone through various stages so far, such as giving up working and social activities and has experienced frustration due to his structured dependency. Nevertheless, he decided to explore a new appearance and to pursue a new lifestyle in order to feel young again. His intentions are an example of what Gilleard and Higgs (2000) have called 'cultures of ageing', which referred to contexts pertaining to older people for new actions that were constructed in societies. Older people may take on new actions in accordance with the new values that have been constructed for them. For example, old people may focus on treating wrinkles, travelling to new countries, or trying out new activities. Indeed, whole industries have been built, or expanded upon, to satisfy the needs of the elderly. It is, however, a mutual process; the new value of older age has not been constructed in a vacuum but, rather, due to increased needs, which resulted from the older baby boomers in the 2010s. Gilleard and Higgs (2000, p. 2) titled their book *Cultures of Ageing: Self, Citizen and the Body* in order 'to give priority to the role of culture in shaping the experience and expression of ageing'. David wants to wear jeans and exercise, thereby imbuing his body with these two symbols of youth. Gilleard and Higgs explained that people use tools or technologies to construct and reconstruct their bodies in accordance with what is fashionable or valuable to society.

David's plans, and the culture of ageing he is entering into, are on a par with the term 'life-course', which refers to the continuing changes in people's social status as they grow older, highlighting that age is not a static phenomenon but a very dynamic lifelong process (Bury, 2000, p. 90). When they become older, people participate in different domains in life, and they may change social roles or differentiate the intensity of their participation. In other words, life is not staged; instead, it is a course with changing opportunities and contexts for social activity. To further illustrate the changing nature of social roles, Macmillan and Copher (2005, p. 859) used the terms 'trajectories' and 'transitions'. Trajectories are the stages of social participation in society (i.e., adulthood, employment, retirement). Transitions are chronological periods between one trajectory and another. For example, the periods from childhood to adulthood or from working to retirement both represent transitions. This means that the change from one stage to another is not sudden or abrupt but rather it is mediated by transitional periods during which individuals do not have clear roles and social expectations might be blurred. To touch on the term life-course, David states that he is not old, which means that, to David, age is not staged in distinct periods but is a continuing process and experience. According to him, he is now entering into a new trajectory, that of being young again. David's words also point towards another direction; that is, old age is not a natural context but a social construction.

AGE AS A SOCIAL CONSTRUCT

David states that he does not feel old, despite the fact that he is 80 years old. This is a very interesting statement, which might possibly be challenged by the majority of younger people. Basically, David challenges the definition of old age. What is old age, anyway? Laslett (1987) explained that old age has been defined on the basis of life expectancy in modern societies. In other words, old age is reached around the time that the age of death is defined by a society. This means that there is no objective or natural definition of old age. Laslett carried on clarifying that, on the basis of life expectancy, four ages have been constructed. The first age refers to the early age of dependency and socialisation in people's lives. The second age, perhaps the longest, relates to the financial capacity and activity of people. The third age occurs after having achieved the basis of cultural goals and is the period before the fourth age, when the person becomes fragile and dependent again due to ill health. However, these definitions were nothing more than a social fabric and modernisation has contributed to defining people who had reached the age of life expectancy as aged, frail, and worth excluding from social and economic activities.

Fennell et al. (1994) maintained that new technologies, industrialisation, and the social importance of education have placed older people, who used to be considered a reliable source of information in pre-modern societies, in a social position of less value and importance. In conclusion, the increase in life expectancy, the growth of older populations, the need to provide power to and create job opportunities for younger people, advancements in technology, and the education of younger people have dramatically changed the symbolism of elderly people from powerful and important to powerless and a burden on the younger generations. To make symbolisms a reality, modern societies have drawn boundaries around ages. They have used the pension age (usually 65) and life expectancy to define a group of people who meet these criteria as old. Old then leads to implications such as exclusion from the labour market, decrease in income, and so forth.

FURTHER DEVELOPMENTS

Unfortunately, David cannot fulfil his newly set goal of changing his appearance and lifestyle. His bowel cancer relapsed and metastasised to the liver and pancreas. The prognosis is very poor and Dr Michael Shepard informs David's wife, Mrs Jane Gordon, accordingly. David may be moved to a hospice. Jane prefers taking care of him and staying close until the end. Dr Shepard is planning to inform David about his condition and that there is nothing else they can do at the hospital to prevent the progression of cancer. Jane asks the doctors not to tell David because David grew up in a culture where the dying were not informed about their imminent death in order not to give up hope. Dr Shepard shows genuine interest to understand more and empathises with

Jane. At the same time, he explains the protocol he has to follow and that there are many patients who want to know whether their condition is terminal or not in order to close any pending issues in their life. Dr Shepard carries on clarifying that he first has to check with David on how much he would like to know and take it from there. Jane likes this approach.

INFORMAL CARE

Jane is an example of an informal caregiver because the care she provides to her husband is not under the auspices of the country's healthcare services. In essence, informal care is provided by individuals that are not under formal institutions of healthcare, such as spouses, parents, and children of people who are in need of care (Yuill et al., 2010; Barrett et al., 2013). The main reason why individuals provide informal care is as a result of kinship ties and obligations and the lack of institutions which could otherwise assume that role. While informal care is largely provided by the family, the traditional concept of family is not the same as it used to be in the past; it has gone through significant changes, such as moving from the extended type to the nuclear, and from the nuclear to a decline in family size, the growth of separated families, different family structures across ethnic groups, and so forth (Yuill et al., 2010). On this note, today, informal care is much harder and more expensive for the carers than it was initially thought to be.

Jane is among the few millions of informal carers in the UK. According to Stevenson (2008), there is a specific distribution of carers based on age and gender. The majority of carers are women; a finding which accords with the cultural values of viewing women as carers of children and the elderly. Interestingly, the majority of carers are between the ages of 35 and 65, reflecting a group of individuals who have either children or older parents who require their support. Informal carers spend specific amounts of time caring for individuals. The time spent is not the same across the spectrum of informal carers; rather, it varies on the basis of class and ethnicity. That is, the higher the social class, the lower the time commitment for care. More specifically, those from higher managerial and professional classes are less likely than those who never worked to spend 50 hours or more per week on care. This class-related time commitment to care possibly has to do with the utilisation of financial and material resources to substitute informal care. That is, people from higher socioeconomic classes are more likely to pay money for services of care for their loved ones.

Ethnicity influences care in different ways. Based on the national statistics, those that are more likely to provide care in general are White British, White Irish, and Indians. These three ethnic groups are more likely to provide care because of possible differences in the age of the population of each ethnic group. For example, there are more elderly White British who are in need of support and care compared to other ethnic groups such as Black Africans. Within ethnic groups, differences have been observed in time commitment for care. Those who are more likely to care are also more likely to spend 50 hours or more per week on care. Other ethnic groups are less likely to commit more time for care due to their increased need to pursue other activities, such as work and financial survival (Stevenson, 2008). Jane is White British, and she is very willing to provide care to her older husband who suffered a heart attack. Though statistics show that the White British are more likely to commit 50 hours or more per week on care, Jane appears to be unwilling or unable to make such a commitment. Her intentions seem to be mediated by her socioeconomic status and occupation. Both she and her husband were teachers and could be classified under the classes 'lower managerial and professional' or 'intermediate' classes, which demonstrated less time commitment than lower classes (Stevenson, 2008, p. 277).

Jane sounds exhausted already. She feels that she cannot adequately fulfil her obligations as David's carer, and she needs to either reduce her time commitments or obtain support from other people or institutions. Jane is among those informal carers who have increased psychological and social needs. In general, informal carers need support to deal with the daily challenges of care, the emotional impact, and their identity. Stevenson (2008) explained that the carers who had more needs were those who had other caring commitments, did not care for a partner or a spouse, did not have strong social networks to draw support from, and suffered ill health. These needs, therefore, reflect broader socioeconomic inequalities in the sense that the carers from the poorer classes would have more unmet needs and would be more likely to require support for caring for their children or parents.

FURTHER DEVELOPMENTS

David finds out about the prognosis. He initially feels angry, but he then changes approach and chooses to die at home surrounded by his loved ones. He wants to close a long-standing dispute he has been having with his brother. A month later he falls unconscious and dies peacefully a week later.

DISCUSS

1. What social aspects about death can you identify?
2. What further information from the literature do you need?

DEATH AND DYING

David's case raises a few social aspects of death. These are social death, sociohistorical changes and the medicalisation of death, awareness context, and good death. Social death refers to a situation where someone cannot communicate with the outside world and needs other people to act on their behalf. For example, people who are in coma, brain dead, or cannot communicate with the outside world could be classified as examples of people who are socially dead (Sweeting and Gilhooly, 1997). The one week during which David had been unconscious could be considered as the period of being socially dead. Social death is more likely to be observed in contemporary times when medical technology may maintain life over a long period of time. Joralemon (2002) stressed the impact of the period between social and biological death which may leave people without a context of externalising intense feelings like what they do after biological death during a funeral. Funerals have social functions, such as intense mourning, perceived closure, place of reference, social event for farewell, which do not seem to apply in the case of social death.

The contemporary phenomenon of social death also reflects changes in the perceptions of death. That is, death used to be a daily experience for people, and it has increasingly become privatised and more scientifically understood (Elias, 1985; Ariès, 1981), resulting in moving death to hospitals and it being scrutinised by biomedicine. Such privatisation and isolation of death and the dying has caused people to be more afraid of death (Bury, 1997). Placing death and the dying under the scrutiny of biomedicine has led to medicalisation of the dying by turning it into a series of pathologies. Such an approach has produced two undesirable phenomena (Illich, 1976, pp. 24, 42). *First*, medical intervention produced 'iatrogenesis', which refers to the health conditions that actually result from medical intervention itself. *Second*, 'cultural iatrogenesis', which refers to biomedicine's intrusion into people's lives and activities, implies that people can no longer manage their pain and suffering, and that biomedicine is required to help them. Put differently, biomedicine did not only intrude into people's bodies, but also into people's social lives and death.

Nowadays, we see more options for the dying patient, such as a hospice or return home as a way to de-medicalise death and the dying (Seale, 1998). David's case is an example of such de-medicalisation as he was provided with all information he chose to have and given options about where to go for care. The concept of de-medicalisation has been revisited recently by Norman and Tesser (2019) by using Kuehlein et al.'s (2010) term 'quaternary prevention' to call for the need to de-medicalise and in order to avoid overdiagnosis and overtreatment. In essence Norman and Tesser's clockwise approach involved taking all necessary actions in the following order: to cure, to detect a health condition early, to reduce the impact, and to promote wellbeing. Martins et al. (2019) tried to improve Norman and Tesser's approach by clarifying that the order does not really matter, and that de-medicalisation should happen in any stage patients find themselves in.

David's case is also an example of the concept of 'aware contexts'. Although the term was used in the 1960s by Glaser and Strauss (1964, p. 670), it has been relevant in recent times. Glaser and Strauss talked about four awareness contexts regarding disclosure of imminent death. *First*, there was the 'closed awareness', in which health professionals did not inform the patient about the imminent death as they thought that the patient did not want to know about it. Closed awareness also functions well for staff that might not want to be faced with emotionally loaded situations that are difficult to handle. *Second*, 'suspicion awareness' occurred when the patient believed that death was coming and when medical staff may have known about it but were not certain. *Third*, through 'mutual pretence', the patient knew that something serious was going on but both sides (the patient and the medical staff) did not openly discuss the matter. Glaser and Strauss named the fourth context 'open awareness', that is, medical staff clearly informed the patient that death was imminent. Seale et al. (1998) found that closed awareness was practised in the past, but open awareness is more likely to be practised today. However, Field and Copp (1999) maintained that open awareness was not a given but was conditional, depending on the situation. Nowadays, patient autonomy is a priority and telling patients about the prognosis of their condition is informed by protocols whereby patients are informed on the basis of how much they would like to know (Silverman, Kurtz, and Draper, 2016).

Dr Shepard followed the protocol as he checked about how much David would like to know, and he demonstrated cultural competence by acknowledging Jane's concerns (see Chapter 1 for more information about Cultural Competence). David chose to learn everything about prognosis and as a result he had the opportunity to die at home and close a long-standing family dispute over a past misunderstanding with his brother. Such an approach reflects the concept of good death as used by Kellehear (1990). Kellehear outlined five defining features of a 'good death'. *First*, the patient knows about the imminent death in order to be able to take any actions regarding their remaining lifetime. *Second*, the dying person needs to make some preparations, such as resolving any pending family issues or disputes. *Third*, the patient might wish to finalise certain public matters, such as the preparation or finalisation of a will or ensuring that their next of kin will be looked after. *Fourth*, the patient needs to withdraw from the workplace smoothly. *Finally*, open awareness and a 'good death' offer the dying person the opportunity to say goodbye to their loved ones.

REFERENCES

Ahlskog JE, Geda YE, Graff-Radford NR, Petersen, RC. Physical exercise as a preventive or disease-modifying treatment of dementia and brain aging. In *Mayo Clinic Proceedings* (Vol. 86, No. 9, pp. 876–884). Elsevier; 2011.

Antczak R, Zaidi A. Risk of poverty among older people in EU countries. *CESifo DICE Report* 2016; 14(1): 37-46.

Age UK; 2016. Available at: annual_review_2016_2017.pdf (ageuk.org.uk).

Aries P. *The Hour of Our Death*. London: Allen Lane; 1981.

Barrett P, Hale B, Butler M. *Family Care and Social Capital: Transitions in Informal Care*. New York: Springer; 2013.

Burholt V, Winter B, Aartsen M, Constantinou C, Dahlberg L, Feliciano V, ... Waldegrave C. A critical review and development of a conceptual model of exclusion from social relations for older people. *Eur. J Ageing*. 2020; 17(1): 3–19.

Bury M. Health, ageing and the lifecourse. In: Williams S, Gabe J, Calnan M, editors. *Health, Medicine and Society: Key Theories, Future Agendas*, pp. 87–106. London: Routledge; 2000.

Bury M. *Health and Illness in a Changing Society*. London: Routledge; 1997.

Elias N. *The Loneliness of the Dying*. Oxford: Blackwell; 1985.

Fennell G, Phillipson C, Evers H. *The Sociology of Old Age*. Milton Keynes: Open University Press; 1994.

Field D, Copp G. Communication and awareness about dying in the 1990s. *Palliat Med*. 1999; 13(6): 459–468.

Fried LP, Carlson MC, Freedman MM, Frick KD, Glass TA, Hill J, McGill S, Rebok GW, Seeman T, Tielsch J, Wasik BA, Zeger S. A social model for health promotion for an aging population: Initial evidence on the Experience Corps model. *J Urban Health*. 2004; 81(1): 64–78.

Glaser BG, Strauss AL. Awareness contexts and social interaction. *Am Sociol Rev*. 1964; 49(5): 669–79.

Giddens A. *Sociology*. 5th ed. Cambridge: Polity Press; 2006.

Gilleard CJ, Higgs P. *Cultures of Ageing: Self, Citizen and the Body*. Harlow: Prentice Hall; 2000.

Hall-Lande JA, Eisenberg ME, Christenson SL, Neumark-Sztainer D. Social isolation, psychological health, and protective factors in adolescence. *Adolescence.* 2007; 42(166): 265–88.

Harris DK. *The Sociology of Ageing.* 3rd ed. Lanham, MD: Rowman & Littlefield Publishers; 2007.

Higgs P. Later life, health and society. In: Scambler G, editor. *Sociology as Applied to Medicine*, pp. 176–92. London: Saunders Elsevier; 2008.

Illich I. *Limits to Medicine, Medical Nemesis: The Exploration of Health.* Harmondsworth: Penguin; 1976.

Joralemon D. Reading futility: Reflections on a biomedical concept. *Camb Q Healthc Ethics.* 2002; 11(2): 127–133.

Kellehear A. *Dying of Cancer: The Final Year of Life.* London: Harwood Academic Publishers; 1990.

Kuehlein T, Sghedoni D, Visentin G, Gérvas J, Jamoulle M. Quaternary prevention: A task of the general practitioner. *Primary Care.* 2010; 10(18): 350–54.

Laslett P. The emergence of the third age. *Ageing Soc.* 1987; 7(2): 133–60.

Macmillan R, Copher R. Families in the life course: Interdependency of roles, role configurations, and pathways. *J Marriage Fam.* 2005; 67(4): 858–79.

Martins C, Godycki-Cwirko M, Heleno B, Brodersen J. Quaternary prevention: An evidence-based concept aiming to protect patients from medical harm. *Br J Gen Pract.* 2019; 69(689): 614.

Marx I, Van den Bosch K. *How Poverty Differs from Inequality: On Poverty Measurement in an Enlarged EU Context: Conventional and Alternative Approaches.* Belgium: Centre for Social Policy, University of Antwerp; 2000. Available at: http://epp.eurostat.ec.europa.eu/portal/page/portal/conferences /documents/34th_ceies_seminar_documents/34th%20CEIES%20Seminar/1.1% 20%20I.%20MARX.PDF.

Moody HR. Ageing, meaning and the allocation of resources. *Ageing Soc.* 1995; 15(2): 163–84.

Norman AH, Tesser CD. Quaternary prevention: A balanced approach to demedicalisation. *Br J Gen Pract.* 2019; 69(678): 28.

Silverman J, Kurtz S, Draper J. *Skills for Communicating with Patients.* Boca Raton: CRC Press; 2016.

Seale C. *Constructing Death: The Sociology of Dying and Bereavement.* Cambridge: Cambridge University Press; 1998.

Stevenson F. Community care and informal caring. In: Scambler G, editor. *Sociology as Applied to Medicine*, pp. 193–205. London: Saunders Elsevier; 2008.

Sweeting H, Gilhooly M. Dementia and the phenomenon of social death. *Sociol Health Illn.* 1997; 19(1): 93–117.

Taylor S, Field D. *Sociology of Health and Health Care.* 4th ed. Singapore: Blackwell Publishing; 2007.

Townsend P. The structured dependency of the elderly: A creation of social policy in the twentieth century. *Ageing Soc.* 1981; 1(1): 5–28.

Xu J, Kochanek KD, Murphy SL. Death: Final data from 2007. National Vital Statistics Report. *US Department of Health and Human Services.* 2010; 58(19): 1–135.

Yuill C, Crinson I, Duncan E. *Key Concepts in Health Studies.* London: Sage; 2010.

CHAPTER 10

Digital health

······································

ABSTRACT

John Goodman is 60 years old, and his recent blood test showed that he has prediabetes. He has been advised by his doctor to cut down added sugar, reduce the amount of carbs he consumes during the week, and exercise regularly. John is a university professor and is concerned that he will not be able to keep pace with all these expectations due to his busy schedule but also the COVID-19 pandemic and any future lockdowns which might make his life even busier. He is informed by his doctor to look into the possibility of using e-health or digital health technology to help him overcome the challenges and keep him focused on improving his health status. This chapter aims to help healthcare students and practitioners understand the social aspects of digital health and any structural influences on use and access by patients.

LEARNING OBJECTIVES

- Explain what the term digital health means.
- Identify and describe specific types of digital health.
- Describe the effectiveness of digital health.
- Explain people's acceptability of new technology.
- Outline the structural impact on digital health.

DOI: 10.1201/9781003256687-11

> *Note: Think about or discuss the questions that are in the boxes before you continue reading through the chapter.*

SCENARIO

John Goodman visited his GP to discuss his recent blood results. All were fine except his blood glucose which was 115 mg/dL, indicating that he has prediabetes with increased chances of developing type II diabetes in the next couple of years if he does not make lifestyle changes and monitor his glucose level with follow-up blood tests in due course. John is particularly concerned because he has to take actions during the COVID-19 pandemic and during possible upcoming lockdowns. He is a university professor with a very busy schedule, and he does not think he can focus on monitoring his health and blood glucose.

DISCUSS

1. Why does John think that he cannot focus on monitoring his health?
2. What could support him to achieve his goal of monitoring his health and prevent type II diabetes?

FURTHER DEVELOPMENTS

Dr Julia Tanner: Good morning, Mr Goodman. How do you feel today?

John: I am fine, thank you! I have come to discuss my blood results. The lab sent me the results, it seems that my blood sugar is high.

Dr Julia: Let me check the results. You are right. They are all fine except blood glucose which is outside the reference range. It should be below 100 mg/dL, but it is 115 mg/dL. And this is the second time in three months, from what I see from your notes. Are you familiar with what this type of result means?

John: Well, I know that it indicates prediabetes. What I do not know is what I have to do now.

Dr Julia: We could discuss some options like lifestyle changes, such as diet and exercise.

John: I am not sure what that means. I have a balanced diet and I go cycling sometimes.

Dr Julia: Would you like me to talk a little bit more about some options.

John: Sure.

Dr Julia: We can discuss and agree on what works for you. The thing is that you have diabetes in your family, your mother was diagnosed with diabetes when she was 53. This increases your vulnerability in addition to ageing.

John: Yes, I know.

Dr Julia: It would be good to reduce or cut down the amount of added sugar you consume. Also, your carb intake should be limited, while some fruits should be avoided. Systematic exercise, preferably on a daily basis, would be beneficial. Walking, for example, works well with reducing glucose, in case you do not want to do anything more rigorous.

John: Doctor, I can exercise more, I can reduce carbs. I am not sure about sweets, though. I really like them.

Dr Julia: I see, there are many people who like sweets, including myself, and I understand how cutting down can be difficult. However, you can take this step by step. I will refer you to a nutrition specialist who works with patients with diabetes to help you adjust your eating habits in a way that works for you. Is this OK with you?

John: Thank you, Doctor, this sounds like a good plan. Is there anything else I can do to have a lifestyle schedule and better monitor my glucose levels?

Dr Julia: Some of my patients have used digital technology.

John: Digital technology? What does that mean?

Dr Julia: There are apps which help patients remember things, make their own lifestyle schedule, adhere to therapy, get scores and feedback, etc.

Dr Julia: You look worried, Mr Goodman. Could you please tell me what your concerns are?

John: Your suggestion caught me by surprise, and I have many questions, Doctor. Where can I find this technology? How do I know it can help me? Is it one device, is it more?

Dr Julia: I can give you a website to check what is available and see what can fit your schedule and your needs. This is just a suggestion to try in case you strongly feel you cannot keep pace with your busy lifestyle and at the same time keep an eye on your health and blood glucose. When you find something that you think could be helpful, please let me know. We have to make sure that it can really help you.

John: Thank you, Doctor, I will.

DISCUSS

1. How could technology be used in the case of John?
2. What is digital health and how could it help John?

DEFINITION OF DIGITAL HEALTH

Henwood and Marent (2019) explained that defining digital health is not a straightforward task, largely because it is a broad term which encompasses many aspects of health, technology, and social behaviour. Lupton (2018, p. 1) attempted a comprehensive definition by defining digital health as

> a wide range of technologies directed at delivering healthcare, providing information to lay people and helping them share their experiences of health and illness, training and educating healthcare professionals, helping people with chronic illnesses to engage in self-care and encouraging others to engage in activities to promote their health and well-being and avoid illness.

In an earlier work, Lupton (2014) explained that there were millions of apps designed for smartphones, tablets, and other devices that people engaged with well. Lupton carried on presenting the historical context of developing mobile apps and digital health. More specifically, she explained that the development of the world wide web provided massive access to information about health and constructed settings of discussions. Therefore, from a situation where only healthcare professionals and students had access to medical information we moved to the 'e-patients' (Lupton, 2014, p. 608) where patients learn how to take control over their health. The emergence of the world wide web placed the grounds for the development of apps regarding health, health management, and prevention, resulting in thousands of such health-related apps. Although the quality of these apps and accuracy of information have been debated, both lay people and healthcare professionals use them (Lupton, 2014).

Lupton clarified that these technologies were not objective tools. Instead, they were created by human beings within a specific economic and sociocultural context and should be approached more critically by scientists and lay people. For example, apps about reproduction use language and information that are gendered and biased in favour of male dominance. In addition, healthcare apps place particular emphasis on individual understanding of and responsibility for health and illness downplaying or completely overlooking social determinants of health. Interestingly, Henwood and Marent (2019) advised that sociologists focused on both structural and behavioural determinants of health. Within the context of behavioural determinants, technology can be a tool for monitoring individuals' health and causing them to develop a sense of control. However, within the context of structural determinants of health, technology could be understood as a way to control the powerless and direct their frame of thinking and actions. Rich and Miah (2014) maintained that the proliferation of digital technologies has increased the level and degree of surveillance of people's lives.

It seems that there are many healthcare apps for lay people nowadays and John is likely to have many options. In John's case, the use of technology is more relevant to behavioural determinants because he has not been influenced by other social structures affecting the development and management of diabetes (e.g., low socioeconomic status). Instead, it seems that he is more vulnerable because his mother had type II diabetes and behavioural or lifestyle changes could potentially help him to bring his glucose levels back to the normal range.

FURTHER DEVELOPMENTS

John Goodman decided to talk with Dr Julia Tenner on the phone to have his questions addressed.

John: Doctor, I had a look and I am not sure what technology I prefer. I will look into it further and ask again, but for now I have a couple of questions.

John: I am wondering how other people who have used it have accepted digital technology. Also, do we know if such technology has helped people with prediabetes or diabetes?

Dr Julia: Thank you for raising these questions. It is good that you have as much information as possible. There is some evidence to suggest that digital technology has helped patients. However, we have to revisit this when you decide on some options.

John: OK, thank you. Also, my concern is that what is going to happen if we have to go through another lockdown. How am I going to use the technology?

Dr Julia: That I do not know. We can discuss again when you decide which technology you will be using.

DISCUSS

1. How is new technology accepted by people?
2. What factors determine acceptability?
3. How has digital technology been used during the COVID-19 pandemic?
4. Is digital technology effective for the control of diabetes?

ACCEPTABILITY OF NEW TECHNOLOGY

Acceptability of new technology is essential for long-term use of devices by older people. Many studies have illuminated this issue and clarified a number of characteristics and functions of new technology which could potentially cause older people to engage with it well. More specifically, Vassli and Farshchian (2017) and Vandemeulebroucke, de Casterlé, and Gastmans (2017) explained that older people are likely to use technology when it is not intrusive and when they control the technology and not the other way round. Shareef et al. (2020) revealed that older people were keener on a 'boss–employee' relationship with robots whereby they would prefer making all decisions. The above-mentioned studies also highlighted other characteristics, such as privacy and trust. That is, cameras, sensors, or robots intruding in older people's personal space were perceived as important barriers for acceptability and long-term use. Moreover, prior experience with other technology with similar functions was another factor for boosting the use of new devices. So, familiarity and positive experiences with other technologies was very important for older people. Interestingly, older people were not willing to use technology as it would cause them to reduce social interactions with other people and they would be enthusiastic to use technology that would help them to socialise more.

Apart from the sense of control and privacy that older people would like to enjoy, studies indicated that the perceived usefulness of new technology was among the key factors for acceptability. Such perceived usefulness relates to a technology that would satisfy older people's needs (Louie, McColl, and Nejat, 2014), and would improve their health condition (Fischer et al., 2014) and quality of life (Vichitvanichphong et al., 2014). Hawley-Hague et al. (2014) advised that older people would be convinced about technology's usefulness if the technology was reliable and did not fail often.

In addition to perceived usefulness, more studies placed emphasis on the physical and functional characteristics of the technology in order for older people to accept and use it in the long run. Some studies showed that older people would prefer technology with simple functions, a machine-like appearance (instead of human-like appearance), a projecting female voice, and responding and expressing emotions (Fang and Chang, 2016; Broadbent, Stafford, and McDonald, 2009).

Beyond any characteristics and functions of new technology as outlined above, there are some individual characteristics which could potentially affect acceptability by older people. Amaro and Gil (2011) found that age played a role in the sense that the older they were, the less likely to be willing to use new technology. This was because more advanced age was associated with poorer technology literacy, but also with limited capability due to the presence of a limiting condition or comorbidities (Astell, McGrath, and Dove, 2019; Kim et al., 2009). Claes et al. (2015) indicated that the financial cost of new technology could also jeopardise acceptability and long-term use of new technology. Interestingly, Broadbent, Stafford, and MacDonald (2009) maintained that gender shaped older people's understanding of using new technology. That is, women focused on the interactive skills of new technology, whereas men focused on the functions of technology. Fang and Chang's (2016) study showed that men were less likely to accept using technology on the arm and neck, but women did not seem to have an issue with these bodily locations. Also, social reactions on the use of devices were an issue of concern for men but not for women.

Constantinou et al.'s (2021) study concluded that designers of new technology for older people should meet the N-ACT principles in order to ensure acceptability and use in the long run. N-ACT stands for Needs, Adaptability, Control, and Trust. This means that a technology which (a) satisfies older people's needs, (b) is adaptable to people's changing needs and provides personalised care or service, (c) does not take control away from the users, and (d) is reliable and promotes a sense of trust is more likely to be accepted and used. In support, Constantinou et al.'s (2021) piloting of vINCI (Clinically validated Integrated Support for Assistive Care and Lifestyle Improvement: the Human Link) technology which employed three devices (a mobile app, an insole, and a watch) showed that older people accepted this technology well because of the following characteristics: how to use it was easily understood and learned, the devices were comfortable on the body, it was easy to use, it was useful and safe, users had control, technology was familiar, and users continued their lives as normal, as before, with no disruption. Constantinou et al. (2021) expanded their pilot to qualitatively check how two older families accepted the vINCI technology. The in-depth interviews indicated that older people appreciated that the technology was enjoyable, familiar, and gave a sense of purpose and control.

Based on the above, it seems that the answer to John's question about how older people accept technology is not straightforward. It depends on many factors. However, some basic characteristics, such as ease of use, usefulness, maintenance of control, etc., seem to be generally relevant to all new technology tailored for older people. What John also needs to understand better before he decides which technology to use relates to the effectiveness of digital health technology, which is further discussed below.

EFFECTIVENESS OF DIGITAL TECHNOLOGY

A rapid systematic review by Bitar and Alismail (2021, p. 15) shed some light regarding the use of digital health by chronic patients during the COVID-19 pandemic. The objective of the study was to summarise the current status and expert opinions, recommendations, and evidence associated with the use and implementation of digital health for chronic patients during the COVID-19 pandemic. Bitar and Alismail identified 51 studies and eventually reviewed 25 which met their inclusion criteria. They found that e-health, telemedicine, and telehealth have been used for the following reasons: follow-up visits, training, consultations, medications, communications, and caregiver support. For improving the use, the following recommendations have been generated: system integration, remote outpatient care, billing reimbursement, continuity of care, standardised transition process, cost-effectiveness, simplicity, privacy, and data sharing.

John rightly wondered whether digital technology would help him manage glucose levels and prevent type II diabetes developing. Although answering this question safely is a challenge because it depends on the technology that John will be using and the fact that a technology is effective when there is research evidence to compare means between groups and not individuals, some studies indicate that digital technology can work well with the control of glucose levels. Huter et al.'s (2020) scoping review focused on the effectiveness of digital technology for nursing care. They reviewed 121 studies and 31 reviews and found that some studies showed a positive impact, yet the quality of the evidence was not high. They highlighted the importance of more thorough research on specific technology and the use of randomised control trials in order to reach safe conclusions. Puleo et al. (2021) conducted a systematic review on the cost-effectiveness of digital health technology. The 35 studies they reviewed indicated that in general, digital health technology is cost-effective, with positive health outcomes. At the same time, the authors clarified that comparison of the studies included was difficult due to the variety of technologies and methodologies employed; hence, they suggested a more standardised procedure and method for evaluating digital technology.

A systematic review and meta-analysis by Kebede et al. (2018) focused on the effectiveness of digital intervention for improving control of glucose levels among patients with diabetes. The review explored 21 randomised control trials (RCTs) and showed that digital technology was effective in controlling glucose levels among patients with diabetes. Idris et al.'s (2020) study of the effectiveness of a digital lifestyle programme, which participants immersed themselves into and submitted their weights after 6 and 12 months, indicated that the programme significantly improved patients' weight, contributing towards enhancing the management of diabetes. However, the European Association for the Study of Diabetes (EASD) and the American Diabetes Association (ADA) published a common report acknowledging some evidence on the effectiveness of digital technology in managing diabetes but raised a number of issues, including, among others, the need to regulate such technology and patients to discuss thoroughly with their healthcare provider before using specific apps or other relevant devices (Fleming et al., 2020).

This information has given some confidence to John that technology can help. He liked the idea that technology can be a tool under his control. He thought that the use of technology would give him a sense of new purpose. He decided to look into it in order to make sure which technology can better meet his needs and reflect his lifestyle and will discuss again with Dr Julia Tanner in order to make the most appropriate selection.

FURTHER DEVELOPMENTS

John shares his experience of prediabetes and his venture into digital technology with Ala Farid, his female neighbour.

John: Ala, I told you that I was diagnosed with prediabetes. Now I have to be more careful with diet and exercise in order to control my glucose level. It is 115, I have to get it down to 100 or less. I hope I can do it.

Ala: I am sure you will, you are a stubborn boy. [*Laughs*]

John: I know but I cannot help it much with sweets. So, I will use technology, it will be on my phone, like an app, which will help me.

Ala: How can an app help you? What is an app anyway?

John: It is what you get with a smartphone. It can help me have health and lifestyle programmes, reminders, I can set goals, get feedback, and soon. I have not yet found the best one, but I will get there soon. I think you should use it too for your diabetes. I know that it works.

Ala: How much is this technology, John? I do not have much money, you know.

John: I do not know for sure, but it can be costly. I can help you with this if you want to try it.

Ala: Thank you, John. But I need more. I need to know what it is, how I can use it, and so on. I do not even have a smartphone. I think I prefer my pills and my doctor's advice only.

John: I see. Well, I will try it and let you know. You can think about it more later.

DISCUSS

1. What questions can be raised from the dialogue between John and Ala?
2. Can the existing literature provide some insights into these questions?

DIGITAL HEALTH AND INEQUALITIES

What Ala has raised reflects the literature regarding the issue of digital technology and social inequalities well. Social inequalities and the need for structural competence have been presented and discussed in Chapter 6. In general, lower socioeconomic status is associated with ill health, largely due to materialist (i.e., access to resources) and behavioural (i.e., human actions) reasons. Social inequalities also relate to gender (e.g., lower wages), ethnicity (poorer health among members of ethnic minority groups), and age (i.e., older people and social disadvantage). As Rich, Miah, and Lewis (2019) have explained, one government objective was the use of digital health to significantly contribute to reducing social inequalities in health. In fact, there is evidence to suggest that this objective has not been met.

More specifically, Muller, Wachtler, and Lampert (2020) conducted a narrative literature review and found that the majority of studies included in their review discovered an association between digital health interventions and sociodemographic factors. For example, digital technology was largely utilised by younger, educated people with higher income. The authors concluded that there was no evidence indicating that digital health has reduced inequalities. Along similar lines, Sawert and Tuppat (2020) analysed data from more than 5,000 participants and revealed that using digital technology was associated with higher educational levels. George et al. (2018) highlighted the importance of general inequalities in using digital health, asserting that women are placed in a disadvantaged position, while Poole, Ramsawmy, and Banerjee (2021) stressed the digital divide among ethnic minority groups. Interestingly, Henwood and Marent (2019) have talked about the importance of structural factors in shaping inequalities, where factors or forces such as class, gender, and ethnicity influence the course of health outcomes.

John raised valid concerns regarding making lifestyle changes in order to better control his glucose levels. He delved into the possibility of using digital technology to help him better monitor his health. John learned that people are more likely to accept technology and use it in the long run, provided that the technology is easy to use, it is useful, does not take control away from the user, and does not cause the user to change their routine. Research shows that digital technology can be useful for people for monitoring both general health and diabetes control. However, John should discuss any potential technologies with Dr Julia before any final decision is made.

REFERENCES

Amaro F, Gil H. ICT for elderly people: Yes, "They" can! In: *Proceedings of 2011 e-CASE & e-Tech International Conference*; 2011. Available at: https://core.ac.uk/download/pdf/62717788.pdf.

Astell A, McGrath C, Dove E. That's for old so and so's!: Does identity influence older adults' technology adoption decisions? *Ageing Soc.* 2019; 40: 1550–76. https://doi.org/10.1017/S0144686X19000230.

Broadbent E, Stafford R, MacDonald B. Acceptance of healthcare robots for the older population: Review and future directions. *Int J Soc Robot.* 2009; 1(4): 319–30. https://doi.org/10.1007/s12369-009-0030-6.

Claes V, Devriendt E, Tournoy J, Milisen K. Attitudes and perceptions of adults of 60 years and older towards in-home monitoring of the activities of daily living with contactless sensors: An explorative study. *Int J Nurs Stud.* 2015; 52(1): 134–48. https://doi.org/10.1016/j.ijnurstu.2014.05.010.

Constantinou CS, Gurung T, Motamedian H, Mavromoustakis C, Mastorakis G. New ambient assisted living technology: A narrative review. In: Magaia N, Mastorakis G, Mavromoustakis C, Pallis E, Markakis EK, editors. *Intelligent Technologies for Internet of Vehicles*, pp. 487–99. Cham: Springer; 2021.

Constantinou CS, Mavromoustakis C, Philippou A. Piloting the vINCI technology in Cyprus. In: The XIII National Congress of Geriatrics and

Gerontology with International Participation Functional Independence of Older People and Active Longevity. Oct 28-31, Romanian. *J Gerontol Geriatrics*. 2021; 10(1): 31.

Constantinou CS, Mavromoustakis C, Philippou A, Mastorakis G. Piloting intelligent methodologies for assisted living technology through a mixed research approach: The VINCI project in Cyprus. In: Magaia N, Mastorakis G, Mavromoustakis C, Pallis E, Markakis, EK, editors. *Intelligent Technologies for Internet of Vehicles*, pp. 501–11. Cham: Springer; 2021.

Cornejo Müller A, Wachtler B, Lampert T. Digital Divide – Soziale Unterschiede in der Nutzung digitaler Gesundheitsangebote [Digital divide – social inequalities in the utilisation of digital healthcare]. *Bundesgesundheitsblatt – Gesundheitsforschung – Gesundheitsschutz*. 2020; 63(2): 185–91. German. 2021 Aug. Erratum. In: *Bundesgesundheitsblatt – Gesundheitsforschung – Gesundheitsschutz*, 64(8): 1026. https://doi.org/10.1007/s00103-019-03081-y; PMID: 31915863; PMCID: PMC8057990.

Fang Y, Chang C. Users' psychological perception and perceived readability of wearable devices for elderly people. *Behav Inform Technol*. 2016; 35(3): 225–32. https://doi.org/10.1080/0144929X.2015.1114145.

Fischer SH, David D, Crotty BH, Dierks D, Safran C. Acceptance and use of health information technology by community-dwelling elders. *Int J Med Inform*. 2014; 83(9): 624–35. https://doi.org/10.1016/j.ijmedinf.2014.06.005.

Fleming GA, Petrie JR, Bergenstal RM, Holl RW, Peters AL, Heinemann L. Diabetes digital app technology: Benefits, challenges, and recommendations. A consensus report by the European Association for the Study of Diabetes (EASD) and the American Diabetes Association (ADA) Diabetes Technology Working Group. *Diabet Care*. 2020; 43(1): 250–60.

George AS, Morgan R, Larson L, LeFevre A. Gender dynamics in digital health: Overcoming blind spots and biases to seize opportunities and responsibilities for transformative health systems. *J Public Health*. 2018; 40(suppl_2): ii6–ii11. https://doi.org/10.1093/pubmed/fdy180.

Hawley-Hague H, Boulton E, Hall A, Pfeiffer K, Todd C. Older adults' perceptions of technologies aimed at falls prevention, detection or monitoring: A systematic review. *Int J Med Inform*. 2014; 83(6): 416–26. https://doi.org/10.1016/j.ijmedinf.2014.03.002.

Henwood F, Marent B. Understanding digital health: Productive tensions at the intersection of sociology of health and science and technology studies. *Sociol Health Illn*. 2019; 41(Supplement 1): 1–15.

Huter K, Krick T, Domhoff D, Seibert K, Wolf-Ostermann K, Rothgang H. Effectiveness of digital technologies to support nursing care: Results of a scoping review. *J Multidisc Healthcare*. 2020; 13, 1905.

Idris I, Hampton J, Moncrieff F, Whitman M. Effectiveness of a digital lifestyle change program in obese and type 2 diabetes populations: Service evaluation of real-world data. *JMIR Diabetes*. 2020; 5(1): e15189.

Kebede MM, Zeeb H, Peters M, Heise TL, Pischke CR. Effectiveness of digital interventions for improving glycemic control in persons with poorly controlled type 2 diabetes: A systematic review, meta-analysis, and meta-regression analysis. *Diabet Technol Therap*. 2018; 20(11): 767–82.

Kim E-H, Stolyar A, Lober WB, Herbaugh AL, Shinstrom SE, Zierler BK, Soh CB, Kim Y. Challenges to using an electronic personal health record by a low-income elderly population. *J Med Internet Res.* 2009; 11(4): 44. https://doi.org/10.2196/jmir.1256.

Louie W-YG, McColl D, Nejat G. Acceptance and attitudes toward a human-like socially assistive robot by older adults. *Assist Technol.* 2014; 26(3): 140–50. https://doi.org/10.1080/10400435.2013.869703.

Poole L, Ramasawmy M, Banerjee A. Digital first during the COVID-19 pandemic: Does ethnicity matter? *Lancet Public Health.* 2021; 6(9): e628–30.

Puleo V, Gentili A, Failla G, Melnyk A, Di Tanna G, Ricciardi W, Cascini F. Digital health technologies: A systematic review of their cost-effectiveness. *Eur J Public Health.* 2021; 31(Supplement_3): ckab164–273.

Sawert T, Tuppat, J. Social inequality in the digital transformation: Risks and potentials of mobile health technologies for social inequalities in health. *SOEP Papers on Multidisciplinary Panel Data Research 1079, DIW Berlin, the German Socio-economic Panel (SOEP)*; 2020.

Shareef M, Kumar V, Dwivedi Y, Kumar U, Akram M, Raman R. A new health care system enabled by machine intelligence: Elderly people's trust or losing self control. *Technol Forecast Social Change.* 2020; 162: 120334. https://doi.org/10.1016/j.techfore.2020.120334.

Vandemeulebroucke T, de Casterlé BD, Gastmans C. How do older adults experience and perceive socially assistive robots in aged care: A systematic review of qualitative evidence. *Aging Ment Health.* 2017; 22(2): 149–67. https://doi.org/10.1080/13607863.2017.1286455.

Vassli L, Farshchian B. Acceptance of health-related ICT among elderly people living in the community: A systematic review of qualitative evidence. *Int J Hum–Comput Inter.* 2017; 34: 99–116. https://doi.org/10.1080/10447318.2017.1328024.

Vichitvanichphong S, Talaei-Khoei A, Kerr D, Ghapanchi AH. Adoption of assistive technologies for aged care: A realist review of recent studies. In: *Proceedings of 2014 47th Hawaii International Conference on System Sciences*; 2014. Available at: https://ieeexplore.ieee.org/stamp/stamp.jsp?tp=&arnumber=6758941.

Index

Printed in the United States
by Baker & Taylor Publisher Services

Printed in the United States
by Baker & Taylor Publisher Services